Christine M. Houser

Pediatric Infectious Disease

A Practically Painless Review

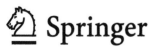 Springer

Christine M. Houser
Department of Emergency Medicine
Erasmus Medical Center
Rotterdam, The Netherlands

ISBN 978-1-4939-1328-2   ISBN 978-1-4939-1329-9 (eBook)
DOI 10.1007/978-1-4939-1329-9
Springer New York Heidelberg Dordrecht London

Library of Congress Control Number: 2014944382

Pediatric Infectious Disease

To my parents, Martin and Cathy, who made this journey possible, to Patrick who travels it with me, and to my wonderful children Tristan, Skyler, Isabelle, Castiel, and Sunderland who have patiently waited during its writing – and are also the most special of all possible reminders of why pediatric medicine is so important.

Important Notice

Medical knowledge and the accepted standards of care change frequently. Conflicts are also found regularly in the information provided by various recognized sources in the medical field. Every effort has been made to ensure that the information contained in this publication is as up to date and accurate as possible. However, the parties involved in the publication of this book and its component parts, including the author, the content reviewers, and the publisher, do not guarantee that the information provided is in every case complete, accurate, or representative of the entire body of knowledge for a topic. We recommend that all readers review the current academic medical literature for any decisions regarding patient care.

Preface

Keeping all of the relevant information at your fingertips in a field as broad as pediatrics is both an important task and quite a lot to manage. Add to that the busy schedule most physicians and physicians-to-be carry of a practice or medical studies, family life, and sundry other personal and professional obligations, and it can be daunting. Whether you would like to keep your knowledge base up to date for your practice, are preparing for the general pediatric board examination or recertification, or are just doing your best to be well prepared for a ward rotation, *Practically Painless Pediatric Infectious Disease* can be an invaluable asset.

This book brings together the information from several major pediatric board review study guides, and more review conferences than any one physician would ever have time to personally attend, for you to review at your own pace. It's important, especially if there isn't a lot of uninterrupted study time available, to find materials that make the study process as efficient and flexible as possible. What makes this book additionally unusual among medical study guides is its design using "bite-sized" chunks of information that can be quickly read and processed. Most information is presented in a question and answer format that improves attention and focus and ultimately learning. Critically important for most in medicine, it also enhances the speed with which the information can be learned.

Because the majority of information is in question and answer (Q & A) format, it is also much easier to use the information in a few minutes of downtime at the hospital or office. You don't need to get deeply into the material to understand what you are reading. Each question and answer is brief – not paragraphs long as is often the case in medical review books – which means that the material can be moved through rapidly, keeping the focus on the most critical information.

At the same time, the items have been written to ensure that they contain the necessary information. Very often, information provided in review books raises as many questions as it answers. This interferes with the study process, because the learner either has to look up the additional information (time loss and hassle) or skip the information entirely – which means not really understanding and learning it. This book keeps answers self-contained, meaning that any needed information is provided either directly in the answer or immediately following it – all without lengthy text.

To provide additional study options, questions and answers are arranged in a simple two-column design, making it possible to easily cover one side and quiz yourself or use the book for quizzing in pairs or study groups.

For a few especially challenging topics, or for the occasional topic that is better presented in a regular text style, a text section has been provided. These sections precede the larger Q & A section for that topic (so, for example, infectious disease text sections will generally precede the question and answer section for infectious disease). It is important to note that when text sections are present, they are not intended as an overview or an introduction to the Q & A section. They are stand-alone topics simply found to be more usefully presented as clearly written and relatively brief text sections.

The materials utilized in *Practically Painless Pediatrics* have been tested by residents and attendings preparing for the general pediatric board examination, or the recertification examination, to ensure that both the approach and content are on target. All content has also been reviewed by attending and specialist pediatricians to ensure its quality and understandability.

If you are using these materials to prepare for an exam, this can be a great opportunity to thoroughly review the many areas involved in pediatric practice and to consolidate and refresh the knowledge developed through the years so far. *Practically Painless Pediatrics* books are available to cover the breadth of the topics included in the General Pediatric Board Examination.

The formats and style in which materials are presented in *Practically Painless Pediatrics* utilize the knowledge gained about learning and memory processes over many years of research into cognitive processing. All of us involved in the process of creating it sincerely hope that you will find the study process a bit less onerous with this format and that it becomes – at least at times – an exciting adventure to refresh or build your knowledge.

Brief Guidance Regarding Use of the Book

Items which appear in **bold** indicate topics known to be frequent board examination content. On occasion, an item's content is known to be very specific to previous board questions. In that case, the item will have "popular exam item" or "item of interest" beneath it.

At times, you will encounter a Q & A item that covers the same content as a previous item. These items are worded differently and often require you to process the information in a somewhat different way, compared to the previous version. This variation in the way questions from particularly challenging or important content areas are asked is not an error or an oversight. It is simply a way to easily and automatically practice the information again. These occasional repeat items are designed to increase the probability that the reader will be able to retrieve the information when it is needed – regardless of how the vignette is presented on the exam or how the patient presents in a clinical setting.

Occasionally, a brand name for a medication or a piece of medical equipment is included in the materials. These are indicated with the trademark symbol (®) and are not meant to indicate an endorsement of, or recommendation to use, that brand name product. Brand names are sometimes included only to make processing of the study items easier, in cases in which the brand name is significantly more recognizable to most physicians than the generic name would be.

The specific word choice used in the text may at times seem informal to the reader and occasionally a bit irreverent. Please rest assured that no disrespect is intended to anyone or any discipline, in any case. The mnemonics or comments provided are only intended to make the material more memorable. The informal wording is often easier to process than the rather complex or unusual wording many of us in the medical field have become accustomed to. That is why rather straightforward wording is sometimes used, even though it may at first seem unsophisticated.

Similarly, visual space is provided on the page, so that the material is not closely crowded together. This improves the ease of using the material for self- or group quizzing and minimizes time potentially wasted identifying which answers belong to which questions.

The reader is encouraged to use the extra space surrounding items to make notes or add comments for himself or herself. Further, the Q & A format is particularly well suited to marking difficult or important items for later review and quizzing. If you are utilizing the book for exam preparation, please consider making a system in advance to indicate which items you'd like to return to, which items have already been repeatedly reviewed, and which items do not require further review. This not only makes the study process more efficient and less frustrating, but it can also offer a handy way to know which items are most important for last-minute review – frequently a very difficult "triage" task as the examination time approaches.

Finally, consider switching back and forth between topics under review, to improve processing of new items. Trying to learn and remember many information items on similar topics is often more difficult than breaking the information into chunks by periodically switching to a different topic.

Ultimately, the most important aspect of learning the material needed for board and ward examinations is what we as physicians can bring to our patients – and the amazing gift that patients entrust to us in letting us take an active part in their health. With that focus in mind, the task at hand is not substantially different from what each examination candidate has already done successfully in medical school & in patient care. Keeping that uppermost in our minds, board examination studying should be both a bit less anxiety provoking and a bit more palatable. Seize the opportunity and happy studying to all!

Rotterdam, The Netherlands   Christine M. Houser

About the Author

Dr. Houser completed her medical degree at the Johns Hopkins University School of Medicine, after spending 4 years in graduate training and research in Cognitive Neuropsychology at George Washington University and the National Institutes of Health. Her Master of Philosophy degree work focused on the processes involved in learning and memory, and during this time she was a four-time recipient of training awards from the National Institutes of Health (NIH). Dr. Houser's dual interests in cognition and medicine led her naturally toward teaching and "translational cognitive science"—finding ways to apply the many years of cognitive research findings about learning and memory to how physicians and physicians-in-training might more easily learn and recall the vast quantities of information required for medical studies and practice.

Content Reviewers

For Infectious Disease Prevention Topics

Seth Rakoff-Nahoum, M.D., Ph.D.
Fellow in Infectious Diseases
Boston Children's Hospital
Boston, MA, USA

For General Infectious Disease Topics

Louise Elaine Vaz, M.D., M.P.H.
Clinical Fellow, Pediatric Infectious Diseases
Boston Children's Hospital
Boston, MA, USA

Contents

Chapter 1
Infectious Disease Prevention Question and Answer Items

Many immunoglobulins used in prevention are now synthesized. Which ones come from pooled serum immunoglobulin, instead?
(2)

- Hep A
- Measles

(give in first 6 days post-exposure)

Is there a monoclonal antibody that's helpful with RSV infection?

Yes – palivizumab
(only used for sickest infants & those with congenital heart disease)

Are there any indications for giving palivizumab (RSV IG) prophylactically?

Yes – infants with

1. **Chronic lung disease**
2. **Prematurity <28 weeks gestation**
3. **Birth between 29–32 weeks gestation & less than 6 months old at start of RSV season**

If RSV IG is started prophylactically, how long should it be continued?

Until infant is 12 months old *and* **RSV season is completed**

(If they turn 12 months during the season, you don't stop it until the season is over)

How common is it for patients to have bad reactions to IVIG?

Not common

If a patient anaphylaxes to IVIG, what underlying immune problem do they probably have?

IgA deficiency

© Springer Science+Business Media New York 2015
C.M. Houser, *Pediatric Infectious Disease: A Practically Painless Review*,
DOI 10.1007/978-1-4939-1329-9_1

What IVIG complication is common in very small patients, especially?

Fluid overload

Most of the time, preemies get their immunization at the regular chronological age. When should immunizations be deferred?
(2 reasons)

1. Medically unstable
2. Inadequate muscle mass to receive immunization (less than 1,500 g)

Is it alright to give a reduced or a divided dose of pertussis vaccine?

No

Why is acellular pertussis a better vaccine than whole cell?

Fewer side effects, but close to the same efficacy

Why do we try to avoid giving more tetanus shots than necessary?

Increased (local) hypersensitivity reactions

At what age are children considered to be at high risk for pneumococcus?

Age 2–5 years

If a child missed his pneumococcal vaccination series, and doesn't present until age 3 years, what should you do about the immunization?

**Start it late
(still in the high-risk age group, until age 5 years)**

If a child aged 2–5 years presents who has not received pneumococcal vaccination, or didn't complete the series of early immunizations, how many pneumococcal vaccine doses should you give?

Just 1

(patients with high-risk conditions, such as sickle cell, may be given one or two doses)

Which pediatric patients are considered "high risk" for pneumococcus, based on other medical conditions?
(4 groups)

Immunocompromised –

- **Sickle cell or other patients with subnormal splenic function**
- **HIV infected**
- **Other – diabetes, chemo, transplant, etc.**

Chronic lung or heart disease

CSF leaks

Cochlear implants

How many types of pneumococcus does the basic childhood immunization cover? (the conjugate vaccine)

Thirteen
(the first vaccine version covered 7 types – it has been replaced)

What is the basic childhood immunization called?

PCV13 –
Brand name Prevnar®

(PCV stands for pneumococcal conjugate vaccine)

How many types of pneumococcal diseases does the polysaccharide vaccine address?

23

(known as PPSV23)

(PPSV stands for pneumococcal polysaccharide vaccine)

Which children get the vaccine for the 23 types of pneumococcus?

>2 years old & high risk

Is there a reason that the polysaccharide vaccine for pneumococcus can't be used for children less than 2 years old?

Yes –
doesn't stimulate an immune response

Which kids qualify for an extra dose of pneumococcal vaccine in the "low-risk" ages from 6 to 18 years?

Kids with high-risk medical conditions who have not previously received the PCV13 vaccine – *even if they did previously receive PCV7 or PPSV23*

What is the protocol for immunizing children with the polysaccharide pneumococcal vaccine?

First immunization after 2nd birthday – One more 5 years later for children with splenic dysfunction & immunocompromise

The "regular" pneumococcal vaccine, PCV13, *cannot* be combined with which other vaccines?

PPSV23 (wait at least 8 weeks after the last PCV13 is given to give PPSV23, if indicated)

&

Meningococcal vaccine
(aka MCV4)

For an asplenic child, which takes priority, immunizing for pneumococcus or immunizing for meningococcus?

Pneumococcus –
It is the more likely problem

At what age can meningococcal vaccine be given?	**9 months for Menactra™ [aka MCV4-D]**
	&
	2 years for Menveo™ [aka MCV4-CRM]
	(Recent change: The FDA has approved Menveo for children as young as 2 months in August 2013, if indicated for travel, etc. This will likely take a year or two to be reflected in board exam questions.)

What is the main shortcoming of the meningococcal vaccine?

30 % of the US cases are type B – the vaccine doesn't cover it

When should the meningococcal vaccine be routinely given?

Age 11 (roughly) & again at age 16–18

Which kids are at highest risk to develop meningococcus?

1. **No spleen**
2. **Complement deficiency (C3 or terminal complement)**
3. **Dorm-style living (including military recruits)**
4. **Travel in endemic area**

Generally, oral polio vaccine should not be used. What are the rare circumstances in which you might choose it?
(2)

1. Outbreaks – useful for mass immunization
2. Incompletely immunized child traveling to an epidemic area

What are the two big problems with oral polio vaccination?

1. **GI shedding can produce disease in non-immune household contacts**
2. **Occasionally causes paralytic polio**

What does the influenza vaccine protect you from?

Most popular A and B strains for each year *(reformulated each year!)*

How many immunizations are normally required for influenza immunity?

One each year *(assuming the vaccine covers the influenza circulating)*

In children less than 9 years old, the influenza vaccine is not as effective as it is in older individuals. How should these young children be vaccinated?

Two doses 1 month apart – just the first year they receive it

Does influenza vaccination have any significant complications?	No
When should you give influenza vaccine?	**October–November (ideally)** *(okay to give until the END of flu season, however, if not given earlier)*
Which kids are at high risk for bad influenza for pulmonary reasons?	**Asthma & chronic pulmonary problems**
Patients taking long-term aspirin therapy should have influenza vaccine. Why?	Greater risk for complications (e.g., Reye's syndrome)
Do metabolic disorders qualify you as high risk for influenza?	Yup
Which patients are eligible to receive Hep A vaccine?	**> 1 year old**
Which patients should definitely receive Hep A vaccination? **(4)**	1. **Chronic liver disease (prevent another insult to the liver)** 2. **Receiving clotting factor concentrates (for clotting factor disorder)** 3. **Living in an endemic state (11 western US states have endemic rates)** 4. **Travel to endemic area**
What is the link between adoption & hepatitis A?	**Children arriving from countries where Hep A is common frequently bring it to their new home – best to immunize close contacts of newly arrived children**
Bites from which types of animals mean that you definitely need to consider rabies prophylaxis?	**Bats and carnivorous mammals**
Which mammal groups do NOT transmit rabies? **(2)**	**Rodents & lagomorphs (lagomorphs are rabbits & hares)**

Can you catch rabies when the nice doggie licks you?

Yes – if there is an area of broken skin (abrasions that you might not notice *do count*!)

If the patient develops rabies, how can this be treated?

**It can't –
That's why we are so careful with prophylaxis**

(Coma protocols show some promise, but virtually all patients die if not immunized)

If you've been in an enclosed space with a bat or animal that might have rabies, are you at risk if the animal never touched you?

Yes – mucous membrane and conjunctival exposure can produce rabies, and breathing droplet of infected urine also seems to cause disease

(& sometimes a scratch isn't so obvious …)

If you think you might have been exposed to rabies, what should you do before you go to the ER?

Very thorough soap & water wash (reduces infection rate dramatically)

Injuries in what location tend to produce clinical rabies the fastest?

Head & neck
(short distance to reach to the CNS)

A squirrel has bitten your patient. Is rabies prophylaxis an issue?

No – that's a rodent

If rabies prophylaxis is needed, what should you give?

Both immunoglobulin & vaccine

- Ig as much as possible around the site of the injury
- Vaccine elsewhere (usually deltoid)

Why must you avoid giving vaccines & immunoglobulin in the same area of the body, at the same time?

They are likely to bind each other, making both useless to the patient

When traveling, patients are at highest risk for rabies exposure from which animals?

DOGS & bats

Rabies is VERY prevalent in dogs in many parts of the world & travelers are at high risk!

If your patient's possible rabies exposure occurred more than a week before they present to you, should you still consider rabies prophylaxis?

YES –
The incubation time is quite variable so it is worth a try, given the dismal treatment options!

If you have a patient at high-risk of contracting rabies (say, an avid spelunker), what should you recommend?

Vaccination
(follow-up vaccine still needed if exposed, but just a booster)

Animals with which sorts of behavior are most worrisome for transmitting rabies?

Unusual (unprovoked) aggression

&

Lethargic/generally ill animals

What is the best way to determine whether the exposure animal has rabies or not?

Sacrifice the animal & check its brain

In what circumstances can you wait to immunize against rabies, even if the immunization status of the animal (against rabies) is not known?
(4)

Well-appearing animal
Behavior normal or provoked
Low risk of rabies in the animal population
Animal can be observed for signs of illness for at least 10 days

When are children at highest risk for developing infections in the childcare setting?

When they've just started in daycare

Which patient group is most likely to develop acute otitis media when they have a respiratory infection?

Young infants

Does having children in daycare increase the overall number of infections in the community?

Yes

Why are children at increased risk of acquiring antibiotic-resistant infections in daycare?

Contact with many children receiving antibiotics (especially in the winter)

What is the main factor in preventing spread of disease in child care settings?

Caregiver's hygiene practices
(mainly hand washing!)

Should children with chronic Hep B or HIV infection be excluded from child care settings?	**No**
If a child has CMV infection, should he/she stay home until it resolves?	No – it is extremely common in the general population, and a very mild illness
If a kid has a rash, but no fever or change in behavior, can he/she still go to daycare?	**Yes**
If a child develops meningococcus, contacts in daycare or preschool should be prophylaxed. How many days back should you go, in terms of giving prophylaxis for contacts?	**Seven!** **(1 week)**
If a possibly non-immune person is exposed to pertussis, how long do you need to wait to know whether he/she will develop whooping cough?	21 days (the cough lasts for weeks – so does the incubation)
Should school contacts get prophylaxis, if a student comes down with pertussis?	**No (just household and childcare contacts)**
Pertussis outbreaks have been a problem in recent years. What change in immunization protocol addresses this problem?	Addition of a pertussis immunization with tetanus in adolescence
If an HIV+ child bites another child at daycare, what should you do?	**Post-exposure testing, and consider prophylaxis** **If the bite drew blood, prophylaxis is definitely needed**
If a Hep B-positive child bites a child who is not immune, what should you do?	**Give Hep B vaccine and immunoglobulin**
If a disease is spread via suspended particles (airborne), then what is needed to isolate that patient?	**Negative pressure ventilation in the room (+ private room and masks for visitors)**

Which relatively common diseases require airborne precautions?	**TB** **Measles** **Varicella** **Disseminated zoster** <u>T</u>o <u>B</u>e <u>VA</u>ry <u>Disseminated</u> you need to be a <u>Measley</u> (small) particle
It is much more common for infections to be spread in droplets, rather than airborne. What does droplet transmission mean?	The organism is in droplets which can't stay in the air for more than three feet
What are appropriate precautions for droplet-borne diseases?	**Mask if going close to patient** **Private room**
Which commonly encountered infectious agents are droplet-borne? (4)	*N. meningitides* **URIs** **Group A strep** **Pertussis**
How are most nosocomial infections spread?	Contact
Which fungus is known to travel through ventilation systems very successfully?	*Aspergillus*
RSV is droplet & contact spread. In addition to droplet & contact precautions, what other strategy is very effective to prevent spread of the infection?	**Cohort staff and patients** **(Put all of the RSV together!)**
Why would preemies born before 28 weeks gestation (or less than 1,000 g) be more vulnerable to varicella than term babies?	**Mom's IG is mainly transmitted after 28 weeks**
How long is airborne transmission of measles a concern?	Until 4 days after the rash develops
How long do you need to maintain droplet precautions for pertussis?	**5 days after you start treatment**

Which children with TB infection are contagious?

Only those with the cavitary or the laryngeal form

(laryngeal is fairly rare – develops either by direct infection from sputum, or hematogenous spread)

Do most children have cavitary TB?

No

If an adolescent develops TB, is he/she likely to be contagious?

Yes – adolescent TB is the same as adult TB – they cough and spread it

It is standard of care to give the influenza vaccine to which pediatric age group (even if the patient is perfectly healthy)?

6–23-month-olds

In which parts of the USA is hepatitis A immunization routinely given?

It is currently recommended for all children at age 1 year, and for older children living in states with high endemic rates, travel to endemic areas, or risk factors for Hep A

(By 2010, at least 10 states had mandated this vaccine for select groups of people, from food handlers to daycare attendees to kindergarten students)

In general, which vaccines can be administered together, without losing safety or efficacy?

Any of them
(must use separate sites, though)

(very similar vaccines, such as the two forms of pneumococcal vaccine, should be separated in time IF both are being administered)

While it is fine to give vaccines at the same time, in separate sites, what is the special rule about varicella vaccine and the MMR?

If varicella vaccine is given *before* the MMR, you must wait 28 days to give the MMR

Note: This is true for any live vaccines given in succession

If you have the option to give a combination vaccine or individual vaccines, which will the board expect you to do?

Combination
(reduce the number of "shots," when possible)

If the schedule of routine immunizations has been interrupted, how much time must pass for you to be required to start the series over?	**It is _never_ necessary to start the series over**
Which immunizations may need extra doses if the immunization schedule has been interrupted?	**None**
If there has been a long lapse since the last immunizations were given, and the child is significantly behind schedule, what should you do?	**Use an accelerated schedule**
If you are not sure whether a child has received prior immunizations, and there is no timely way to find out, what should you do?	**Give them anyway (assume that they were not given)**
Is it important to be consistent about the brand of vaccine you are using for a particular immunization?	No – except for DTaP (because different brands use different strains & safety/efficacy data has not been collected for mixed types of immunization)
If you have started a DTaP series, and the correct line of vaccine is not currently available, what should you do?	Give the one you have (it's better to have a nonmatching vaccine than not to have it at all)
Is there a link between HepB vaccination and multiple sclerosis?	**No**
Are certain vaccinations linked to autism?	**No**
Which vaccinations are recommended at age 11–12 years?	**Td (booster) HPV (if female) Meningococcus & any "leftover" immunizations that were missed**
If a family refuses to give their children immunizations, what is the best way to handle the situation? (2 parts)	**1. Keep them in your practice (so you can …) 2. Continue to educate the family**

What is the National Childhood Vaccine Injury Act?	Legislation that mandates what you must do each time you give an immunization
What are the four core items a physician must do, according to the National Childhood Vaccine Injury Act?	1. **Give the vaccine "information sheet"** 2. **Discuss risks/benefits** 3. **Document vaccine & lot given in med record** 4. **Report adverse events**
If a patient has an egg allergy, and you give the MMR, what is likely to happen?	**Significant, but manageable, local reaction**
If there is a moderate or severe infection going on when you would like to give an immunization, what are you supposed to do?	**Defer immunization**
If a child has a congenital immune disorder, is it alright to give him/her live vaccines?	**No**
HIV patients are an exception to the rule that immunocompromised patients cannot receive live vaccines. Which live vaccines is it alright to give HIV patients, and under what circumstances?	**MMR & varicella –** **If they are not severely immunocompromised or very symptomatic** **(patient should have >15 % of expected T cell count to receive the varicella vaccine)**
If a patient is receiving chemotherapy, is it alright to give live vaccines?	**No**
What is the importance of knowing whether your patient received gamma globulin, in terms of the patient's immunization schedule?	**Gamma globulin (IVIG) makes certain vaccines much less effective:** **Wait 8 months after IVIG before giving the MMR of VZV immunizations**
In the MMR, which component is most sensitive to interference from other immune molecules?	Measles

If a patient is in the midst of a short course of steroids (<2 mg/kg/day), should immunization with live vaccines be deferred until the steroid course is completed?

No – okay as long as it is short-term and low dose (<2 mg/kg/day)

(short term means <14 days)

**Are there any vaccines that can't be given
to a breastfeeding mother?**

No

If a patient has a cold, should vaccinations be deferred?

No

If a patient has a febrile illness, with fever <40.5 °C and nontoxic appearance, should vaccinations be deferred?

No

If a patient has been ill enough to be given antibiotics for an infection, should you defer vaccination until the antibiotic course is completed?

No

If a child has been exposed to measles, and he/she is not immune, what should you do?

Give measles immunoglobulin – you have 6 days to do it

If a patient is not immune to hepatitis A, and you are concerned about possible future exposure, what are your options?

1. Vaccine (two doses needed for lasting immunity, but the first shot is protective after 4 weeks)
2. Post-exposure IgG
3. Pre-exposure IgG

Which vaccines are live?

Think of an <u>MOB</u> of <u>V</u>accines acting lively –

**MMR
Oral polio
BCG (for TB)
Varicella**

As you learn the recommended vaccination protocols, what should you remember about how they apply to babies born prematurely?

Use the same ages for their immunizations

(unless they are medically unstable or <1,500 g when you would normally give the vaccine)

All childhood immunizations are given IM except for which three? (all given SQ instead)

<u>V</u>aricella
<u>O</u>ral Polio (of course)
<u>M</u>MR

Mnemonic:
VAry Odd In Muscle!

Which live vaccine(s) should be given to a certain population of immunocompromised patients?

MMR & varicella to HIV infected (if not symptomatic at the time of vaccination, and for varicella CD4 T count ≥15 %)

If an HIV patient is seriously immunocompromised, would you still give the MMR?

No – the risks & benefits shift in that case to not giving it

Is oral polio virus still used in the USA? **No**

MMR and varicella are both live vaccines, like oral polio. Is it okay to give those vaccines if the child lives with someone who is immunocompromised?

Yes – they're not communicable or shed in any way (with oral polio vaccine, viable virus is shed in the stool)

Occasionally, a child who has been immunized for varicella develops a varicella-type rash about 1 month later. Why is this important?

Must avoid contact with immunocompromised people (this mild varicella infection *can* be transmitted to others)

Which two live vaccines are sometimes given for children who are traveling (not given routinely)?

Typhoid (oral)
&
Yellow fever

Is there any vaccine that is recommended to be given *at birth*, at least in certain circumstances?

Yes – Hep B if mom is surface antigen positive or her status is not known

If the Hep B vaccination needs to be given at birth, how long do you have to give it?

<u>**12 h**</u>

If Mom is Hep B surface antigen positive, what should you give the newborn, in addition to Hep B vaccination?

Hep B Ig (immediately)

If mom's Hep B status was unknown at the time of delivery, but the screen done at delivery comes up Hep B+, how long do you have to give immune globulin? (or should you give it empirically at birth when the mom's status is unknown?)	• Don't give empirically (expensive) if >2,000 g, • Give empirically if <2,000 g • You have 1 week to give it
When do kids born to Hep B-negative moms get their first Hep B immunization?	First 2 months of life (anytime okay in the 2-month interval)
How many shots are in the Hep B vaccination series?	Three
How long do you need to wait after the first Hep B vaccination before giving the second one?	1 month
If you miss a shot in the Hep B series, how long do you have before you need to start the series all over?	Doesn't matter – still works even if it's given years late
What is the youngest age at which it's alright to give the third dose of Hep B vaccine?	6 months
What is special about when you give the third dose of Hep B vaccine, in relation to the other two doses?	Must be <u>2 months</u> after <u>2nd</u> dose, and <u>4 months</u> after the <u>1st</u> dose
What are two good, typical, regimens for the Hep B immunization series?	• Birth, 1 month, 6 months • 2 months, 4 months, 6 months
When are the majority of childhood immunizations given?	• 2–6 months old • 3 sets of 4 vaccines –
What is generally given?	DTaP IPV (polio) PCV (*S. pneumo*) Hib (also Hep B, depending on regimen)
When are the three sets of four immunizations usually given?	2, 4, and 6 months

Of the group of immunizations given three times, ages 2–6 months, which ones require a 4th dose?	<u>All</u>
Are any live vaccines given in the first 12 months of life?	No
Which vaccines are due (along with cake and balloons!) for the infant's first birthday?	• **4th dose of Hib & PCV** • **Varicella and MMR, and sometimes DTaP**
What is the rule for when you can give the final dose of DTaP?	6 months after the third one is given (anytime after 12 months, if the first three were given on schedule)
What "booster shots" are needed when kids are ready to start kindergarten (about age 5 years)?	<u>D</u>TaP <u>I</u>PV <u>M</u>MR **(Kindergarteners who don't get their boosters are DIM because they miss school when sick!)**
Should hepatitis A vaccination be routinely given?	No – it is given for travel to endemic areas and in selected US regions (2 shots – 6 months in between)
Which immunization is *routinely* given at age 11 years?	**Tetanus (Td)** **(and often meningococcus & HPV)**
Which immunizations can be "caught up" at age 11 years, if they were missed?	**Hep B** **MMR** **Varicella**
Is HPV vaccine only for females?	No, the quadrivalent vaccine is also useful to decrease anogenital cancers in males & can be offered
Must you give HPV vaccination before sexual activity begins?	No – Recommended until 26 years old, because exposure to all 4 HPV types in the vaccine has probably not occurred
How often are tetanus boosters (Td) given routinely, without any injury?	Every 10 years

What is the significance of calling the tetanus immunization for older people Td, and the one for younger people DT (DTaP)?

Vaccines listed as DT have 10 times the amount of diphtheria toxoid as do the Td vaccines
(same stuff, just different proportions)

At what point do you switch to Td, rather than a DT vaccine?

> 7 years old

(after that, there is a much greater probability of bad reactions to the diphtheria part, so the amount is kept low)

Egg allergy means that your patient may have a serious reaction to which vaccine?

Influenza
(NOT MMR!)

If a patient has had an anaphylactic reaction to eggs, what do you need to do in terms of still providing him/ her with the necessary immunizations?

Do skin testing to determine whether vaccine can be safely given.

Is it alright to give Hep B immunization to an adolescent who is pregnant?

Yes – just avoid the live vaccines

It is *not* okay to give a vaccine if _____?
(the sole general reason)

**The last time the child had it →
anaphylaxis**

Is hepatitis B virus found in the breast milk of Hep B-positive moms?

Yes

Is it okay for hepatitis B-positive mothers to breast feed?

Yes –
No increase in risk of transmission

Chapter 2
Selected Infectious Disease Topics

Funny Bacteria Overview
(Unfortunately, Not Really Funny, Just Peculiar!)

First, to briefly review, bacteria come in three general groups: **cocci**, **bacilli**, and **spirochetes**. Bacteria usually have both a cell wall and a cell membrane.

Orientation to Bacteria

Spirochetes are strange, spiral bacteria. *The thinnest bacteria are the spirochetes –* often they cannot be seen with a regular microscope at all. (That is why "dark-field microscopy" is needed to make them show up.)

Some bacteria are variable in shape, and those are called **pleiomorphic**.

Mycoplasma is the smallest bacteria, and is about the same size as the largest viruses. *Mycoplasma is also unusual because it lacks a cell wall –* these bacteria only have a cell membrane. It is the smallest independently living organism we know of.

Gram-positive bacteria have a much thicker cell wall than gram negatives do. **Gram negatives** have a different composition for the outer portion of their membrane, and a space between the inner and outer layer where their resistance enzymes often live. Gram negatives also have endotoxin on their cell wall.

Mycobacteria are **acid-fast**. They will not gram stain, because their cell wall contains special lipids called **mycolic acids**.

Outside the cell wall, many bacteria have other specialized structures. One important structure shared by many bacteria is the **glycocalyx coat (slime layer)** which allows the bacteria to adhere to various surfaces. Other bacteria have **capsules of polysaccharide** which make it hard for phagocytes to eat them. This

© Springer Science+Business Media New York 2015
C.M. Houser, *Pediatric Infectious Disease: A Practically Painless Review*,
DOI 10.1007/978-1-4939-1329-9_2

makes them much more virulent than the same bacteria without a capsule. Typical examples of encapsulated bacteria are *Streptococcus pneumoniae* and *Neisseria* species.

In addition to the enzymes contained in the periplasmic space between the cell wall layers of gram-negative bacteria, bacteria often have **plasmids** of double-stranded DNA in their cytoplasm. These plasmids replicate independently, and often provide resistance to various drugs or environmental situations.

Transposons, or genes that jump about on various bits of DNA in the cell, sometimes also provide coding for important resistance mechanisms. Transposons do not replicate independently – they are replicated whenever the DNA to which they are attached at that moment decides to replicate.

Peculiar Types of Bacteria

Mycobacteria (*M. tuberculosis & leprae* + *M. marinum & scrofulaceum, MAI & Kansasii*)

Mycobacteria are proper bacteria, but they are neither gram positive nor negative. They are, of course, acid-fast (due to the high lipid content of their cell wall – mycolic acids). The three types that cause disease in normal hosts are *M. tuberculosis*, *M. bovis* (comes from infected unpasteurized milk), and *M. leprae* (leprosy).

The "atypical" mycobacteria generally cause clinical disease in immunocompromised hosts. Most cause tuberculosis-like illness (organisms *M. kansasii*, *M. avium-intracellulare*). An important exception is *M. avium* intracellular (MAI), which causes cervical lymphadenitis in healthy kids, without immunocompromise.

Atypical mycobacteria that cause disease in normal hosts are *M. marinum* (swimming pool/fish tank granuloma – can be salt or freshwater) and *M. scrofulaceum* (one of the causes of "scrofula" – mycobacterial cervical adenitis – *M. tuberculosis* can also cause scrofula).

Actinomycetes (Actinomyces & Nocardia)

The two general groups of actinomycetes are *Actinomyces* and *Nocardia* species. These are true bacteria, but very strange because they form long, branching filaments that look like fungal hyphae. Nocardia is weakly acid-fast.

Actinomyces is part of the normal oral flora, and sometimes causes orofacial abscesses with the famous "sulfur granules."

Nocardia is found in the environment, mainly in soil. It causes pulmonary infection in immunocompromised hosts, with the special features of abscesses and draining sinus tracts! In normal hosts, one can get pustular lesions at the site of bacterial entry.

Mycoplasma
Very small bacteria with a cell membrane only (no wall). The lack of a wall explains why beta-lactams and cephalosporins can't touch them! Their shape is variable, due to their flexible cell membrane.

The cold agglutinin test is often positive (although not diagnostic) for mycoplasma infection. A positive cold agglutinin test means that the patient has IgM antibodies to type O blood, which will agglutinate the RBCs at cold temperatures (4 °C), but not at body temperature. Official diagnosis is via serology or PCR from nasopharyngeal swabs (now available at many centers).

Spirochetes (*Treponema, Borrelia, Leptospira*)
These guys look like very skinny corkscrews. They come in three varieties: *Treponema* (syphilis, and several tropical diseases such as yaws and pinta – all killed by PCN), *Borrelia* (Lyme disease and relapsing fever), and *Leptospira* (leptospirosis). Both *Leptospira* and *Treponema* species are too thin to be seen with light microscopy. All species are flexible and motile.

Treponema – Interestingly, there are nonpathogenic species that are part of the normal flora of human mucous membranes. Treponema cannot be cultured, but infection can be confirmed with a variety of tests (nonspecific ones are called "reagins," whereas specific ones are "treponemal").

Borrelia – The most irregularly shaped spirochete, they are "loosely coiled." Borrelia can be seen with light microscopy (Giemsa stain). *Borrelia burgdorferi* (Lyme disease) is, of course, transmitted by ticks. The other Borrelias are transmitted by human body lice and "soft ticks." Rodents and other small mammals are the main reservoir for all of the *Borrelia* species. Treat with doxycycline or amoxicillin.

In relapsing fever (caused by *Borrelia recurrentis* – sounds like "recurring," and *Borrelia hermsii* – the two "i's" tell you that it keeps coming back) patients get ill, then develop appropriate antibodies, and get better. Unfortunately, though, as the first infection is getting started, these Borrelias develop different versions of themselves, by creating several versions of their surface markers. This means that although the antibodies have eradicated one variety of Borrelia, and the patient gets better, another type is just waiting to get started. That's why the patient has "relapsing fever." Typically, there will be between three and ten relapses, with well periods between each, before the fevers stop recurring.

Leptospira – tightly coiled and very skinny: It is found in the urine of many types of infected mammals, and transmitted to humans through mucosa & skin abrasions – *usually when the human enters or contacts water contaminated with leptospira.* Dogs are the most important reservoir in the USA, although *rodents are the most important reservoir worldwide.* It is especially likely following swimming after a significant rain, when more infected urine has just been swept into the water. PCN kills it, as does doxycycline.

Chlamydophila (formerly *Chlamydia*)

Chlamydia have strange cell walls – they are rigid and similar to gram-negative cell walls, but have their own unique makeup. *Chlamydia cannot make the energy they need to grow – that is why they are obligate intracellular parasites.* They prefer to invade epithelial cells of mucous membranes in various parts of the body. In addition to serovars L1, L2, and L3 which cause lymphogranuloma venereum, there are also serovars type A – L. Some of those serovars cause mainly ocular Chlamydia, while others cause infection of the genital tract and related structures. *C. pneumoniae* and psittaci mainly affect the lungs.

Chlamydial infections can be identified by inspecting infected cells and recognizing the *cytoplasmic* inclusion bodies, or through laboratory testing. Serological testing can be effective for diagnosing *C. pneumoniae* and psittacosis, but is not helpful for trachomatis (too many people have been exposed to trachomatis to make serological testing useful). ELISA, DNA probes, and PCR of urine or infected exudates are used for definitive diagnosis of trachomatis, and the organism can also be cultured with appropriate support.

Treatment is with tetracyclines or macrolides.

Rickettsiae (the Final Strange One! Typhus, Spotted Fevers, Q Fever, Ehrlichiosis)

All rickettsiae are transmitted to humans by arthropod vectors except one. What is it?

> *Coxiella burnetii* (Q fever) – aerosol transmission

Which rickettsial illness is mainly associated with wars & poverty, and is nearly always spread human to human (humans are the main reservoir)?

> Epidemic or louse-borne typhus – *R. prowazekii*
> Spread by the human louse *Pediculus humanus humanus*.
> (Despite the name, it does not have to occur in large numbers of people at the same time. It is generally a quite severe & sometimes fatal illness.)

. . . but is also seen in the USA due to contact with *flying squirrels*???

> Yes, flying squirrels. They are the only other known vertebrate reservoir. Contact usually involves close contact with the squirrel itself, or with squirrel nests.
> (There are other typhus forms like endemic and scrub typhus, not common in the USA, which are usually due to contact with animal vectors.)

Rickettsiae normally inhabit endothelial cells of blood vessels. Which one targets a different tissue?

> Q fever – lungs

Which rickettsial illness does not cause a rash?

> Q fever – its main interest isn't vessels, and damage to vessels is what causes rickettsial rashes.

Rickettsiae are very short rods – they can be seen with light microscopy, but just barely. *Like Chlamydia they don't have enough energy to reproduce unless they are in a host cell. This makes them obligate intracellular parasites (and still bacteria).*

The *Weil-Felix test* helps to identify patients suffering from rickettsial diseases. It is an agglutination test based on the existence of rickettsial antibodies in the patient's serum. It is not used now in the USA (because it is not very reliable), but can still appear on boards exams. Serological tests of immunofluorescence or ELISA testing are usually used for diagnosis.

Rickettsiae like to live in the endothelium of vessels. That is why you find them causing vasculitis, in most cases.

Typhus should not be confused with *typhoid*! Typhoid is infection with *Salmonella typhi*. Typhoid is mainly a GI infection. Typhus, on the other hand, is caused by several rickettsial species (*Rickettsia typhi, prowazekii, and tsutsugamushi* – the main type in the USA is prowazekii). Typhus begins like a bad case of influenza (fever, chills, headache, etc.). It then develops into a maculopapular rash, with accompanying meningoencephalitis. If untreated, peripheral vascular collapse or bacterial pneumonia often causes death after a few weeks.

Epidemic typhus is transmitted by the bite of the human body louse, and humans are the typical reservoir for the rickettsial organism. In the USA, flying squirrels are also a reservoir, and contact with them is sometimes implicated.
Endemic typhus is transmitted to humans by fleas, and has a rodent reservoir.

Treatment:
All rickettsial diseases are treated with tetracyclines, but chloramphenicol is a backup (not really available anymore, but good to know for board exams).

Prevention:
Vaccines are available for typhus, when needed, and also for Q fever (although the Q fever vaccine is not available in the USA). Q fever vaccine is recommended for people who are routinely exposed to the animals most likely to transmit it (shepherds, farm workers, veterinarians, lab personnel, and slaughterhouse workers). Remember that the highest concentration of *Coxiella burnetii* is found in the *placentas* of infected animals. A typical history is a farmer tending to the births of his or her livestock, or a family visiting the very recent birth of some livestock or domestic animals, or spreading of manure (containing the decaying material loaded with bacteria).

Parasite Classification

Protozoa, roundworms, and flat worms are the types of parasites. (Of course, being a parasite also means they live in, or on, a host – and do harm to the host.)

Protozoa

>Amebas, Flagellates, Sporozoans Ciliates

>| Amebas: | *Entamoeba histolytica & Naegleria fowleri* |
>| Flagellates: | Giardia, Trichomonas, Trypanosomes, Leishmania |
>| Sporozoans: | Plasmodium, Cryptosporidium, Toxoplasma |
>| Ciliates: | *Balantidium coli* |

Roundworms = Nematodes

>Ascaris and Enterobius (enterobius=pin worms), trichuris (whip worm), Trichinella, Strongyloides, Ancylostoma & Necator (hook worm), Wuchereria, *Loa loa*, Onchocerca, Dracunculus

Flatworms

>Trematodes: *Schistosomes, Clonorchis, Paragonimus*
>(Trematode = fluke)

>Cestodes: *Taenia, Echinococcus, Diphyllobothrium*
>(Cestode = tapeworm)

Helminth means worm – roundworms and flat worms are both helminthes.

Miliary Tuberculosis

Miliary tuberculosis occurs when massive bacteremia from a tuberculosis infection results in infection of multiple internal organs (at least two). The organs most often affected are the lungs, spleen, liver, and bone marrow. (Meningitis and peritonitis are also possibilities.)

Miliary tuberculosis usually develops 2–6 months after the initial infection, for those patients who are destined to develop it. *Most patients who develop miliary TB, though, do not have a known history of the disease.*

This disorder most commonly occurs in TB-infected infants and young children, although it is seen occasionally in adults.

The onset is usually slow, although it can be sudden. There are two phases to the illness. Initially, the patient experiences fatigue and malaise, and then later develops high fever, lymphadenopathy, and hepatosplenomegaly. Over a period of several weeks, the lungs usually fill with foci of tubercular infection, called "tubers." This can result in respiratory distress and pneumothoraces.

The CXR will be normal in the early phases of miliary tuberculosis. Elderly patients often die of the disease before the chest X-ray shows any related abnormalities.

The most important factor in diagnosing miliary TB in children is a history of exposure to a tuberculosis infected adult. Thirty percent of children with miliary tuberculosis will not test positive for TB. Alternatively, if an affected area, such as a lymph node, can be identified it can be biopsied for a definitive diagnosis.

Children respond well to treatment for miliary TB. Full recovery may take months, but they feel better within 2 weeks. The prognosis is less good for adults with miliary disease but improves if diagnosis and administration of the appropriate treatment are rapid.

Lymphocytic Choriomeningitis

On the pediatric boards, tends to be presented as a zoonosis from pet hamsters. Mice are also a source. It is an arenavirus.

Main point – In humans, it causes aseptic meningitis (rare cause).

Spread by – mice (and sometimes hamster) urine or feces.

Human-to-human spread? – No.

Main reason scientists are interested in this virus – because it is a good example of **"immunopathogenesis."** In other words, it is the immune system response that determines whether this virus makes the animal sick.

If a mouse has incompetent (ineffective) humoral & cellular immunity, and catches the virus, the virus can replicate like crazy, and the mouse does fine.

On the other hand, if the mouse has competent humoral immunity (antibody production) but not cellular immunity, and catches the virus, the mouse will be fine except that over time it will develop glomerulonephritis due to immune-complex deposition.

If the mouse is fully immunocompetent, though, it gets very sick very fast and often dies. Transplacentally infected mice have chronic lifelong infection, and pass the virus along to other mice.

Chapter 3
General Infectious Disease Question and Answer Items

When is toxoplasmosis typically transmitted to a fetus (under what conditions)?	When the mother has a primary infection
Immunosuppressed patients sometimes experience reactivation of toxoplasmosis infections. Can congenital toxoplasmosis develop during reactivations?	**Yes**
Transmission of toxoplasmosis is most likely in what part of pregnancy?	Late (14 % first trimester, 60 % third trimester)
Congenital toxoplasmosis is generally most severe when acquired during what trimester?	The first (the earlier the infection, the greater the effect, in general)
Is congenital toxoplasmosis usually evident at birth?	**No – at least 75 % are asymptomatic**
What two organs does congenital toxoplasmosis prefer?	Eyes & CNS
Is congenital toxoplasmosis more or less common in preemies?	More
What is the "classic triad" of symptomatic congenital toxoplasmosis?	1. Obstructive hydrocephalus 2. Intracranial calcifications 3. Chorioretinitis (white dots on retinal exam)

© Springer Science+Business Media New York 2015
C.M. Houser, *Pediatric Infectious Disease: A Practically Painless Review*,
DOI 10.1007/978-1-4939-1329-9_3

What is the main natural reservoir for toxoplasmosis?

Cats

In addition to cat feces, where else might someone encounter toxoplasmosis?

1. Undercooked meat (especially pork) and eggs
2. Unpasteurized milk
3. Transfusions (of blood products including WBCs)

When an adult is infected with toxoplasmosis, how do they present?
(2 possibilities)

1. Usually they don't present – it's subclinical
2. Nonspecific illness with fever, lymphadenopathy, +/– rash

What is the most typical outcome of congenital toxoplasmosis infection

Visual impairment & learning disabilities (presenting months to years later)

In addition to nonspecific findings such as lymphadenopathy, fever, and hepatosplenomegaly, what other findings/signs are likely in infants with obvious congenital toxoplasmosis?
(4 categories)

1. Chorioretinitis
2. Seizures
3. Microcephaly or hydrocephaly
4. Eye abnormalities (cataracts, microphthalmos, optic atrophy, glaucoma, etc.)

What tests should be done to confirm suspected congenital toxoplasmosis?
(3)

1. **Serum** (for IgM)
2. **CSF**
3. **Head CT**
(for calcifications)

If a neonate has congenital toxoplasmosis, what do you expect to see in the CSF?
(3)

1. **High protein**
2. **Pleocytosis**
3. **Xanthochromia**

How is congenital toxoplasmosis usually treated? (asymptomatic)

12 months of: pyrimethamine + sulfadiazine + leucovorin

(some use spiramycin in the last 6 months)

How long should an apparently healthy infant be treated for congenital toxo if his/her mother is known to have contracted the disease during pregnancy?

4 weeks
(then confirm the diagnosis)

If a pregnant woman is known to be toxo infected (primary or recurrent), should she be treated?

Yes –
Reduces risk of fetal infection or loss

What anti-inflammatory is sometimes given to infants with symptomatic toxoplasmosis?

Steroids

During treatment, infants with toxo must be monitored for medication side effects with what three tests?
How often?

1. **CBC**
2. **Platelets**
3. **UA**

- **Every week**

During what part of pregnancy is rubella infection most likely to affect a fetus?

U shaped probability –
either early or late in gestation is bad

What kind of virus is rubella?

RNA

What is the natural reservoir for rubella?

Non-immunized humans *only*

If a child seems to have mononucleosis, but is negative for EBV, what is a likely cause?

CMV

What are latex agglutination tests used for?

(same infectious diseases as CIE or counter-immunoelectrophoresis testing)

Partially treated infections

(looks for bacterial cell wall components)

What organisms can a latex agglutination test identify?

Grp B strep
H. flu
N. meningitidis
Strep pneumoniae

Which patients are most likely to have false-positive latex agglutination tests?
(2)

Hib vaccinated

&

Those infected with certain *E. coli* types

What medications can be used to eliminate the carrier state of diphtheria?

Erythromycin or penicillin

Diphtheria vaccination protects a patient from what aspect of the infection?

The carrier state

Although *Pneumocystis carinii/jiroveci* (PCP) is an opportunistic infection, it is often seen in children without a known history of immunocompromise. Why?

It tends to be the first opportunistic infection

If a child is known to be at risk for PCP, what medication should be started?

Bactrim®

(generic is TMP/SMX)

In an immunocompromised child with fever & neutropenia, what general categories of antimicrobials will your initial management definitely include?

1. Gram+ antibiotic
2. Gram− antibiotic (e.g., aminoglycoside)
3. Antipseudomonal

If a child presents with atypical tuberculosis, what underlying problem should you consider?

Immunocompromise

Abdominal pain or obstruction + exotic foreign travel or foreign birth = what diagnosis?

Ascaris lumbricoides

(at least think of it)

How is ascaris infection treated?

Albendazole, mebendazole, or ivermectin

"Staccato cough" – first 2 months of life – no fever – tachypnea =

Chlamydial pneumonia

What is the buzzword for *Chlamydia pneumoniae* infection on micro examination?

Intracytoplasmic inclusion bodies

How is chlamydial pneumonia treated?

Erythromycin
(or other macrolide)

Can chlamydial pneumonia be seen in adolescents/adults?

Yes
(it is another atypical along with mycoplasma)

How is chlamydial pneumonia definitely diagnosed?

Immunofluorescent antibodies
Imagine fluorescent pink "Chlams" glowing in the dark

What is the name of the only rickettsial disease that causes pneumonia but <u>no</u> rash?

Q fever

A patient who presents with headache and a rash that moves inward from the extremities may have what serious infectious disease?

RMSF (Rocky Mountain spotted fever)

How is the rash of Rocky Mountain spotted fever described?

Maculopapular –

- **Starts on extremities**
- **Becomes petechial/purpuric**

What is the treatment of choice for RMSF (Rocky Mountain spotted fever)?

Doxycycline (regardless of age!)

Why is it alright to use doxycycline in a child less than 9 years old if you are treating RMSF?

(Cost-benefit)

1. Risk of death vs. risk of tooth staining
2. Tooth staining is unlikely with short-term use anyway

What is a good way to remember the rash pattern for RMSF?

If you were rock climbing in the Rockies, you would probably get some petechiae on your hands & feet

In case of doxycycline allergy, what alternative medication can be used to treat RMSF?

Chloramphenicol

How can CMV be transmitted to a neonate?

(4)

1. Transplacentally with maternal infection (usually primary infection)
2. At delivery with maternal cervical colonization
3. Breast milk
4. Blood transfusion

If a pregnant mother contracts CMV, is she likely to notice the infection?

Usually noticed, but not always reported (nonspecific malaise-type illness)

What percentage of asymptomatically CMV-infected neonates develops serious visual, hearing, or cognitive impairments by age 2 years?

About 10 %

What is "classic CMV inclusion disease?" (6 components – One big thing Two small things Two sensory issues One lab thing)	1. IUGR 2. HSM (with jaundice & high LFTs) 3. Thrombocytopenia 4. Microcephaly 5. Sensorineural hearing deficit 6. Chorioretinitis
How common is congenital CMV infection in the USA?	**1–2 % of births!**
Can a fetus contract CMV from a maternal reactivation of the disease?	Yes, but very rare
What are the significant teratogenic effects of primary rubella infection? (4 groups)	1. CV/heart problems (PDA & pulmonary artery stenosis) 2. Sensorineural hearing loss 3. Cataracts/glaucoma 4. IUGR
What percentage of rubella-exposed infants seems normal at birth?	**>50 %**
Rubella-exposed infants are at risk for late-developing problems in what four organ systems?	1. Special senses (hearing deficit) 2. CNS – (MR, autism, etc.) 3. Endocrine (DM & thyroid dz) 4. Immune system (dyscrasias)
If a pregnant mother contracts CMV, what tends to happen to the fetus even if it does not become infected?	Low birth weight/SGA
CMV is very common in the USA. Its effect in pregnant is unusual, though, because maternal infection during what part of pregnancy most often causes fetal infection?	Equal – It is always about 50 % (for primary infections)
What is the long-term complication rate for infants born with *symptomatic* CMV infection?	**High! 40–90 %**
What is the probability that an infant infected with CMV will be symptomatic?	**10 % are symptomatic**

What intestinal parasite is associated with bloody, mucous-y diarrhea and tenesmus?

Entamoeba histolytica

Eosinophilia is a clue to look for in what type of infection?

Parasitic

What is *toxocara canis* (in very general terms)?

A dog parasite (worm) that sometimes accidentally ends up in a person (wrong host)

What types of problems/symptoms can *toxocara canis* cause?

- Pulmonary wheezing
- GI – hepatomegaly and/or abdominal pain

How can you remember that metronidazole treats *Entamoeba histolytica*?

Picture a "hysterical amoeba" riding the metro to destruction

(another option is tinidazole)

What other parasitic infection featuring bad diarrhea is treatable with metronidazole?

Giardia lamblia

What is the best way to treat scabies in children?

Permethrin cream

How do you identify scabies as the cause of a patient's itching?

Look for long, narrow burrows at edges of clothing and intertriginous areas

How can you differentiate CMV from toxoplasmosis on head CT?

Both cause calcifications but CMV is periventricular (toxo is diffusely spread throughout)

How can you remember that metronidazole (Flagyl®) treats trichomonas?

They are "flagellated" organisms (sounds like Flagyl®!)

If a patient is found to have trichomonas, how many people need to be treated?

The patient & all sexual contacts

Although current literature suggests that this medication is fine in some stages of pregnancy, for the boards, "can you use metronidazole in pregnancy?"

No
(Ob/gyns do use it, though, so don't panic if you see this in real life)

What is the histological/micro buzzword that tells you that a patient has bacterial vaginosis?

"Clue cells"

(Cells that have little bits of stuff hanging from the edges of their membranes)

What kind of discharge is expected with bacterial vaginosis?
(aka "Gardnerella" –
because it is usually the dominant organism)

Thin & gray
(can be copious)

What do you expect to see on exam of a patient with trichomonas?
(**2 "buzz phrases"**)

1. **Strawberry cervix**
2. **Yellow, frothy discharge**

Mnemonic: The little whips make the discharge frothy, and cause petechiae on the cervix (the petechiae are the strawberry seeds)

What is the name of the organism causing "cat scratch fever?"

Bartonella henselae (a bacteria)

How is cat scratch fever usually treated?

Self-limited –
usually supportive care only

If a patient has unusually severe cat scratch fever, or is immunocompromised, how could you try to treat the infection? (which medication?)

Azithromycin

How would you know that a patient's cat scratch fever is unusually severe?
(2 items)

Significant lymphadenopathy (large & painful)

&

Hepatosplenomegaly

What is the buzzword description for Haemophilus influenza on micro examination?

"**Gram-negative pleiomorphic organisms**"

Although *H. flu* is much less common in the USA due to immunization, which populations are likely to get it?

1. Immigrants/
   foreign visitors
2. Unimmunized US children (younger than school aged)

What is the drug of choice for treating *H. flu* infection?

Ceftriaxone

How aggressive are *H. flu* infections in general?

Very aggressive (jump on them! With Ceftriaxone)

H. flu is one significant cause of otitis media. Do immunized children avoid this infection?

No – the vaccine does not prevent the OM infection

(It is non-typeable *H. flu*, not covered by the vaccine)

If a child has had a properly documented pertussis infection, do he/ she still need to be immunized against it?

Yes!
[This is a change – natural immunity is now known to wane in as little as 4 years, so routine immunization is recommended EVEN AFTER a documented infection!]

Does antibiotic treatment help with the coughing of whooping cough?

It may decrease the coughing if started early, before coughing fits begin

Which antibiotics are most recommended for pertussis treatment?

Azithromycin or erythromycin (macrolides)

What alternative antibiotic may be used for pertussis, in those older than 2 months?

Trimethoprim/sulfamethoxazole

In what phase of pertussis infection is it worthwhile to give antibiotics?

The catarrhal (URI) stage

How does erythromycin improve the catarrhal stage of pertussis infection?

It shortens it
(same for the other antibiotic treatment options)

In what other way is antibiotic treatment of pertussis infection helpful?

Decreases communicable period – not communicable 5 days after antibiotics are started!

Elevated WBCs with a lymphocytosis, and a child with a prominent cough, is likely to be what disease?

Pertussis

(usually in an immigrant, foreign visitor, or preschool group)

Bartonella henselae causes what disorder?

Cat scratch fever

What organism causes whooping cough?

Bordetella pertussis

Gram-negative pleiomorphic organisms = what bacteria?

H. flu

What organism is responsible for the H. *flu* type of otitis media?

Non-typeable H. flu

Thin, gray discharge + clue cells = what disorder?

Bacterial vaginosis

Frothy, yellow discharge + strawberry cervix = what disorder?

Trichomonas vaginalis

Contacts of individuals with pertussis need what treatment?

Erythromycin prophylaxis

Should individuals who have been successfully immunized against pertussis still receive prophylactic treatment?

Yes – it prevents spread of the organism (asymptomatic individuals may still spread it)

What two animals are the typical carriers for salmonella?

Chickens

&

Humans

(domesticated turtles can also occasionally be a source)

Vomiting, fever, and bloody loose stools 1–2 days after a group picnic is a likely vignette for what infection?

Salmonella

Should salmonella be routinely treated with antibiotics?

No –
It is likely to cause a carrier state

When might you treat salmonella enteritis with an antibiotic?

Very severe infection/
immuno-compromise

To identify an infant at risk for congenital syphilis, should you test the mother, the infant, or either one?

The mother
(infant serum or cord blood is <u>not</u> sufficient)

If a mother is known to have had syphilis but it was treated prior to pregnancy with erythromycin, is congenital syphilis still a concern?

Yes –
Any non-penicillin treatment regimen is suspect

If an infant is born whose mother's HIV status is unknown, what should you recommend?

HIV testing after counseling + consent of mother (some states allow testing without consent, but the above is preferred)

In which body systems does adenovirus cause infection?	1. Respiratory 2. GI 3. Conjunctivitis/eyes 4. GU
How is the GI version of adenovirus transmitted?	Fecal-oral
How is the respiratory version of adenovirus transmitted?	Contact with infected secretions
What unusual version of adenovirus is sometimes seen in groups, after the individuals go swimming in a poorly chlorinated pool?	**Pharyngoconjunctival fever**
What worrisome, but usually spontaneously resolving, complication is sometimes seen with pharyngoconjunctival fever?	**Corneal opacities**
"Preauricular lymphadenopathy" + conjunctivitis (bilateral) =	**Adenovirus Keratoconjunctivitis** (also sometimes responsible for corneal opacities – self-resolving)
When is respiratory adenovirus most common?	Winter + spring
What treatment is needed for adenovirus infections?	Supportive care (+ isolation of health care workers & school children at home)
What are the symptoms of pharyngoconjunctival fever?	1. **Fever** (it's in the name after all) 2. **Conjunctivis** 3. **Pharyngitis, rhinitis and cervical adenitis**
Why does adenovirus sometimes present as meningitis?	**It sometimes causes meningismus**

What type of infection does adenovirus usually cause?

Respiratory
(10 % of peds respiratory disease is supposedly adenovirus)

What sort of GI symptoms does enteric adenovirus cause?

Watery diarrhea (most common in infants)

When adenovirus causes GU effects, what symptoms or signs are seen?
(3)

Gross hematuria
Dysuria
Frequency (more common in males)

Does adenovirus cause upper or lower respiratory symptoms?

Either

If you want to identify adenovirus as the cause of a child's infection, what body fluids should you send?

Stool and nasopharyngeal swab have the highest yield

(can also attempt to isolate from urine or conjunctival swab)

When adenovirus causes lower respiratory infection, what part of the lungs is most likely to be affected?

The lower lobes

During adenovirus infection, what is a CBC likely to show?

Left shift

+

leukocytosis or leukopenia

Which bacterium causes diphtheria?

Corynebacterium diphtheriae

What is the main buzzword for diphtheria infection?

Gray *pseudomembrane* (in the throat)

What aspect of diphtheria infection causes its associated problems?

The exotoxin it makes

What creates the pseudomembrane in diphtheria infection?

Tissue edema

+

Coagulative necrosis of the mucous membrane

How is diphtheria spread, generally?

Respiratory droplets
(+ sometimes via breaks in skin, conjunctiva, etc.)

During which season do most diphtheria cases occur?

Winter (possibly due to more indoor crowding)

If children or adults are exposed to an active case of diphtheria, but have previously been fully immunized, should anything be done?

Yes –
They require erythromycin or PCN & a booster if the last immunization was >5 years ago

Is diphtheria still endemic in some parts of the world?

Yes –
In most of the developing world

What are the four common forms of diphtheria?

1. **Nasal** (infants, especially)
2. **Pharyngotonsillar**
3. **Laryngeal**
4. **Cutaneous**

Why is cutaneous diphtheria important?

It is a big reservoir for infection in warm climates

How long is the incubation period for diphtheria?

1–6 days

Which type of diphtheria is most dangerous?

Laryngeal
(due to easy compromise of the airway)

Which form of diphtheria is most likely to produce a carrier state?

Nasal

What are the four main factors that determine how severe a particular case of diphtheria is likely to be?

1. **Prior immunization** (less severe)
2. **Virulence** (toxigenic form is worse)
3. **Time to antitoxin** (less is better)
4. **Location of membrane** (laryngeal)

What are the four main complications of diphtheria?

1. Airway obstruction/compromise
2. Myocarditis
3. Renal tubular necrosis
4. Demyelination of motor nerves

What precautions should you take with hospitalized diphtheria patients?

Respiratory isolation until *3 consecutive cultures* from infection sites are negative

What is the mainstay of treatment for diphtheria infection?

Diphtheria antitoxin

What is the only form of diphtheria that can be treated by antibiotics alone (no antitoxin needed)?

Cutaneous

How does laryngeal diphtheria present?

Like croup
(it often develops from the tonsillo-pharyngeal form)

After the symptoms of diphtheria begin, how long is it until pseudomembranes start to form?

1–2 days

Although cardiovascular collapse can occur with diphtheria toxin production, the usual course for diphtheria-induced myocarditis is . . . ?

Spontaneous resolution

What, in general, do the neurological complications of diphtheria consist of?

Demyelination of motor pathways

(mainly oculobulbar,
but can also affect peripheral nerves)

What two factors determine the likelihood of diphtheria complications?

1. interval between symptom onset and antitoxin administration
2. quantity of membranes

How does nasal diphtheria present?

Like a nasal foreign body except bilateral

(initially clear discharge,
then serosanguinous, then smelly mucopurulent)

What happens if you try to remove the pseudomembrane of diphtheria?

It bleeds
(most exudates, etc., do not)

What special finding in the vital signs suggests diphtheria?

Heart rate unexpectedly high for temperature

What unusual effects can diphtheria have on the special senses?

Conjunctivitis

&

Aural diphtheria (otitis externa)

Although diphtheria is a clinical diagnosis, what confirmatory test should be sent?

A culture from the membrane or just below the membrane

How many doses of diphtheria vaccine are needed to immunize a healthy young child?

Five

(roughly:
2 months
4 & 6 months
18 months
4 years)

How is diphtheria immunization different for patients older than 7 years?
(2 ways)

1. *Different vaccine –*
   Td or Tdap (adult type) is given rather than DTaP or DT
2. *Different schedule –*
   Two doses at least 4 weeks apart, then repeat 6 months later

What does the lower-case "d" vs. the capital "D" indicate, in the vaccine name?

The lower-case "d" indicates a reduced dosage diphtheria used in older patients

How is diphtheria treated?

1. **An IV bolus of antitoxin (amount varies)**
2. **14 days of PCN-G, procaine, or E-mycin**

How do people become infected with ascaris?

Fecal-oral ingestion of eggs

What are the main organ systems affected by ascaris?

Pulmonary & GI

The life cycle of ascaris is 2 months long. Where do the worms travel in the body?
(4 phases)

1. **Eggs to gut then to portal venous system**
2. **Pulmonary vessels into alveoli**
3. **Coughed up & swallowed**
4. **Grow to adults in small intestine**

What types of animals can ascaris lumbricoides infect?

Humans only

(*1/4 of the world's population is infected!*)

What problems can ascaris cause in children with abdominal ascaris?
(5 possibilities)

1. Obstruction
2. Malabsorption
3. Growth failure
4. Intussusception
5. Abdominal pain

Where does obstruction due to ascaris occur?	**Ileocecal valve**
What sorts of pulmonary symptoms/signs are seen as ascaris migrates through the lung?	**Fever, cough, dyspnea, & wheezing** (causes an eosinophilic bronchopneumonia)
Will you see infiltrates on CXR during the pulmonary migration of ascaris?	Yes
Are patients with ascaris usually symptomatic?	No – If the infection is only moderate, most are asymptomatic
If a patient is diagnosed with ascaris, what other things should you look for?	Other parasites (often multiple infections)
How is ascaris treated?	A single dose of pyrantel pamoate (alternate regimen for kids older than 2 years: mebendazole for 3 days)
Where does aspergillus usually cause infection?	The lung
Is aspergillus likely to cause infection in HIV+/AIDS patients?	**No** (infection fighting depends on phagocytes, not T-cell immunity, for this bug)
What is the most common form of aspergillus infection? Is it invasive?	• **Aspergilloma (pulmonary fungus ball)** • **No**
Which patients are at risk for invasive aspergillosis?	**Those with neutrophil or macrophage problems** (Including chemo, leukemia, long-term Abx, or steroid use)
Where is aspergillus found, & how is it transmitted?	• Everywhere • Transmitted by lightweight airborne spores

In what ways does aspergillosis affect healthy people?

(2)

Ear & sinus infections in warm, wet regions

&

Allergic bronchopulmonary aspergillosis

What is allergic bronchopulmonary aspergillosis?

Local pulmonary reaction to aspergillus spores trapped in mucus

Which patients are at risk for allergic bronchopulmonary aspergillosis?

Those with chronic respiratory disorders

What are the symptoms of allergic bronchopulmonary aspergillosis?
(2 physical findings)
(1 lab finding)
(1 radiological finding)
(1 icky finding!)

Wheezing
Fever
Eosinophilia
Infiltrates on CXR productive cough
(+ *brown mucous plugs*)

As with most invasive fungal diseases of the immunocompromised, what is the prognosis for disseminated aspergillosis?

Bad –
Amphotericin B

&

Debridement are urgently needed

If an aspergilloma causes symptoms, what symptom is it most likely to cause?

Hemoptysis

Why are the infiltrates seen with allergic aspergillosis "*transient?*"

Because they develop in areas where mucous plugs cause obstruction (if the plug is coughed up, they disappear)

How does "otomycosis" appear on physical exam?

Black spores begin at the TM, & may fill the EAM!
(yuck!)

How does sinusitis from aspergillus present?

Chronic sinusitis that doesn't respond to Abx

What are the two buzzwords for allergic pulmonary aspergillosis?

Transient infiltrates

&

Brown or dark mucous plugs

What lab findings suggest aspergillosis?

1. Elevated Ig E
2. Eosinophilia
3. Branching, septate hyphae

Can the aspergillus species that causes human infection be cultured?

Yes

How is noninvasive aspergillus sinusitis treated?

Surgical drainage/ debridement

Aspergillus otomycosis usually coexists with chronic bacterial otitis. How is it treated?

Debridement & treat the external infection (bacterial)

How do people encounter atypical mycobacteria?

Air, water, meat, & egg products

What are _typical_ mycobacterial infections?

(3)

1. *M. tuberculosis*
2. *M. bovis*
3. *M. leprae*

What are atypical mycobacterial infections?

Any that are not the three typical infections

(Those three are tuberculosis, bovis, & leprae)

What type of infection commonly develops with atypical mycobacterial infection in immunocompetent individuals?

Cervical adenitis in preschoolers (rarely, may also cause otitis or mastoiditis)

What immunocompromised patients are at risk for atypical mycobacterial infection?

HIV (other T-cell disorders do not increase rates of atypical mycobacterial infection)

In what situation might atypical mycobacteria cause a chronic infection of skin, soft tissue, or bone?

Following trauma or surgery

What signs suggest that cervical adenitis is due to atypical mycobacteria?

(3 signs)

1. **Single node or single region of LAD**
2. **No systemic symptoms**
3. **Not warm or tender**

Why is the cervical adenitis of atypical mycobacteria often called a "cold abscess?"	It is literally not warm, as most abscesses would be
How is the diagnosis of atypical mycobacterial infection confirmed?	Culture or micro identification from specimen
What prophylactic medications may be given to HIV+ children to prevent atypical mycobacterial infection?	Azithromycin weekly
How is isolated cervical adenitis due to atypical mycobacterium treated?	**Surgical excision** (usually no meds needed)
Why is draining cervical adenitis due to atypical mycobacterium a bad idea?	**It can produce a chronically draining situation** (unless you excise it after making the diagnosis)
After excising an atypical mycobacterium cervical adenitis, should you follow up with an antibiotic?	**No – but the child should be followed for recurrence for 1 year**
What additional diagnostic should be obtained for patients with atypical mycobacterium infection?	CXR
Fever, malaise, and hemolytic anemia go with what tick-borne illness?	Babesiosis (although most people are actually asymptomatic)
Can babesiosis be transmitted from mother to child in utero?	Yes – but uncommon
The ticks that carry babesiosis are also frequently carrying what other disease?	Lyme
Where in the body does babesiosis live?	Inside the RBC
What patients are at special risk of more severe disease with babesiosis? (4)	1. Extremes of age 2. Immunocompromised 3. No spleen 4. Coinfected with Lyme disease

What very similar syndrome to babesiosis is seen in the Western USA?

WA1 protozoal infection (W – Western, A – American)

Approximately what percentage of babesiosis patients also has Lyme infection?

¼

What is the typical presentation for a patient with symptomatic babesiosis infection?

Systemic symptoms:

1. Intermittent fevers – may be high (40 °C)
2. +/– chills, myalgias, arthralgias

Do babesiosis patients have hepatosplenomegaly?

Sometimes – not reliable

(but the spleen is very important in fighting this infection)

What blood test should you send if you are hoping to identify babesiosis infection?

Thick & thin smear (same as malaria)

What special microscopic appearance is the "buzzword" for babesiosis on the smear?

"Maltese crosses" – due to the characteristic grouping of 4 parasites together

What might the UA of a babesiosis patient show?
(2)

Proteinuria

&

Hemoglobinuria

In addition to anemia, what other CBC abnormalities often occur in babesiosis?
(2)

Thrombocytopenia

&

Lymphocytosis (often atypical)

How are mild or asymptomatic cases of babesiosis treated?

Usually no treatment needed

What stains will usually identify protozoal parasites like babesiosis?
(2)

Giemsa or Wright's

What type of anemia is seen with babesiosis?

Normocytic, normochromic

(Remember, it is an acute, not chronic, problem – no time to change the size of the cells being synthesized)

For patients with significant symptoms of babesiosis, or significant risk factors (asplenic or immunodeficient), how should babesiosis be treated?

7 days of clindamycin or quinine

In rare cases of life-threatening babesiosis, how can the patient be treated?

Exchange transfusion

What are the two most worrisome complications of babesiosis?

1. Hemophagocytic syndrome (progressive pancytopenia & LAD)
2. ARDS-type pulmonary problems (usually occur after treatment has begun)

Can you catch babesiosis more than once?

Yes

How long does a tick need to be attached to transmit babesiosis (or Lyme disease)?

Usually 24 h

(*some medical texts dispute this*)

How does someone get blastomycosis?

Inhalation of spores (from soil)

Is blastomycosis more common in children or adults?

Adults

What are the three forms of blastomycosis infection?

1. Pulmonary
2. Cutaneous
3. Disseminated

What form of blastomycosis is most common in children?

Pulmonary

Although many cases of blastomycosis are asymptomatic or spontaneously resolving, how is it treated when intervention is needed?

Mild-moderate –
Itraconazole or fluconazole
Severe – amphotericin B

(treatment requires at least 6 months)

How is cutaneous blastomycosis acquired?

Usually from the pulmonary tree – sometimes directly through skin inoculation

What types of skin lesions might you see with cutaneous blastomycosis?

Nodules, abscesses, ulcerations

Where in the USA are you most likely to develop blastomycosis?

Central & Southeastern USA

(Blastomyces is present in a variety of other countries, also)

Which neonates are at greatest risk for developing a brain abscess after meningitis?

Those who had gram-negative meningitis

In general, what two organisms are most commonly found in brain abscesses?
      (all ages)

Staph

    &

Strep
(various species)

Abscesses in the frontal lobes of the brain usually develop from what source?

Frontal sinusitis

About what percentage of children with congenital *cyanotic* heart disease will develop a brain abscess?

About 3 % (!)

After having a brain abscess, what proportion of kids will have some long-term neurological problems?

About 1/3

What procedure must <u>not</u> be performed on patients with brain abscesses?

LPs

(it is a space-occupying lesion and there is a risk of herniation)

For patients who can talk, what is the most common complaint associated with a brain abscess?

Headache

Headache +/− fever + a focal neurological complaint =

Brain abscess

Do patients with brain abscesses develop meningismus?

Yes −
About 1/3 will

If CSF were obtained from a brain abscess patient, what would you expect to find?

↑ **protein**
↓ **glucose + pleocytosis**

(no organisms unless the abscess has ruptured)

How are brain abscesses typically treated?

Antibiotics (at least 3 weeks)

+

Surgical excision (if it's a single abscess in an accessible location)

If a patient develops a brain abscess and has no obvious source, what three services need to evaluate the patient for predisposing factors?

1. **Dental**
2. **ENT**
3. **Cardiology**

Breast abscesses in adolescents are likely due to what organisms (in general terms)?

Staph aureus

&

Sexually transmitted diseases (STDs)

How are breast abscesses in adolescents treated?

(3)

1. IV oxacillin or nafcillin, then PO meds (total treatment time of 14 days)
2. I & D
3. Compresses

(all are needed)

Should a breast-feeding adolescent or adult continue breast-feeding if she develops a breast abscess?

Yes, from the unaffected breast

(milk should still be expressed, but discarded, from the affected side)

What is the most common cause of bronchiolitis?

RSV (respiratory syncytial virus)

How is RSV bronchiolitis generally treated?

Supportive care

+

β-adrenergic agent for wheeze

Are bronchodilators, or anti-inflammatories such as steroids, useful in treatment of RSV?

Bronchodilators are often used in hospitalized patients, although it is not clear from data whether it is helpful or not

Steroid use is not supported by available data

Which medication is indicated for treatment of severe RSV cases, although its efficacy is not entirely clear?

Ribavirin – Severe disease and/or high risk for severe disease (e.g., transplant patients)

Most effective if started early!

What medication may be given as prophylaxis against RSV infection, and what kind of treatment is it?	Palivizumab (Synagis®) It is a monoclonal antibody (administered IM once per month during RSV season)
What is usually considered to be "RSV season" in the USA?	November through end of March
Which chronic lung disease patients should receive RSV prophylaxis?	≤2 years old & requiring treatment for the lung problem *within 6 months of the beginning* of RSV season
Which heart patients should receive RSV prophylaxis?	≤2 years old & cyanotic or complicated congenital heart disease
Which three sets of preemies require palivizumab prophylaxis?	• Born ≤28 weeks & ≤12 months old at RSV season start • Born 29–32 weeks & ≤6 months old at RSV season start • Born 32–35 weeks & ≤3 months old at RSV season start
Which children require RSV prophylaxis at any age?	Those with difficulty handling airway secretions
Where might patients encounter brucellosis? **(2)**	**1. Contact with farm animals** **2. Unpasteurized dairy products**
Why is brucellosis sometimes difficult to culture?	**It reproduces *inside* the host's phagocytes**
How long does brucellosis infection usually last?	Less than 3 months
How is brucellosis treated?	TMP/SMX or doxycycline – adding rifampin may decrease relapse rates

Why is it important to complete the antibiotic regimen for brucellosis?	To prevent relapses
For symptomatic patients, what are typical findings of brucellosis?	**Hepatosplenomegaly** + **Lymphadenopathy** (localized infections may be found anywhere, however, including the vertebra)
What type of bacterium is brucellosis?	Gram negative (there are four types of brucellosis)
Brucellosis is well known for its tendency to affect which organ system?	Nearly any of them – Endocarditis, gut complaints, neuropsychiatric effects, joint problems, etc.
Where does campylobacter infection come from?	Domestic & farm animals (meat, unpasteurized milk, contaminated water) + Person to person (fecal-oral)
What are the three forms of campylobacter infection?	1. Systemic 2. Enteritis (ileocolitis) 3. Antral gastritis
What is the most common type of campylobacter infection seen in children?	Inflammatory ileocolitis
What special "after effects" of campylobacter are sometimes seen?	**Postinfectious autoimmune complications**
What postinfectious complications are most common following campylobacter infection?	**1. Guillain-Barre** **2. Reiter syndrome** **3. Reactive arthritis** **4. Erythema nodosum**
When is campylobacter infection most common?	**Summertime** **(unlike most bugs that like the winter)**
Nausea, vomiting, *halitosis*, and crampy epigastric pain suggest what infectious diagnosis?	**Campylobacter gastritis**

Along with *Yersinia enterocolitica*, what is campylobacter known for mimicking?

Appendicitis!
(& sometimes intussusception)

Most patients with campylobacter recover quickly. Which two long-term complications are sometimes seen with campylobacter?

Arthritis

&

Guillain-Barre

Campylobacter is estimated to be responsible for what percentage of the US Guillain-Barre cases?

40 %

Does campylobacter enteritis require treatment?

**No –
It usually resolves in about 5 days**

What is a *typical* presentation of campylobacter enteritis?"

Fever, abdominal pain, bloody or mucous-y diarrhea

Are the animals infected with the various types of campylobacter ill?

No – they are asymptomatic

Should campylobacter *gastritis* be treated?

Yes – if not treated it tends to continue in a chronic phase for months

How can campylobacter be rapidly identified in fresh stool specimens?

The curved rods "dart around"

What is the *gold standard* for identification of campylobacter pylori (the gastritis bug)?

Gastric mucosa biopsy & culture (from the biopsy)

What medication is used to treat campylobacter infections caught early?

Azithromycin (many others are often also effective)

How do most patients acquire campylobacter infection?

Contact with contaminated meat

(*proper cooking does kill it*)

Does campylobacter infection pose any risk to fetuses?

Yes
1. Infected mothers (even if asymptomatic) have more abortions & preterm deliveries
2. Fetal & newborn fatal infection sometimes occurs

Do you need to get rid of your cat if someone in the family develops cat scratch disease?	No – the cat is not likely to carry the bacteria chronically
What is the general appearance of a lymph node infected with *Bartonella henselae*?	1. Central necrotic area 2. Hypertrophied 3. Thickened cortex 4. Pus-filled sinuses
Which cats are most likely to transmit cat scratch disease?	Those less than 1 year old
The most frightening complication of cat scratch disease is encephalitis. What is the typical course of this complication?	• **Develops about 1 month after basic cat scratch disease** • **Sudden onset** • **Coma** • ***Full recovery***
Does cat scratch disease cause a rash?	No – But there may be a papule that changes to a crust at the site of the cat contact
Where will you see lymphadenopathy following cat scratch disease exposure?	The lymph nodes draining that area (*unilateral*)
What percentage of the enlarged lymph nodes of cat scratch disease will form a tract thru the skin?	<50 %
How should you treat a tender, large, cat scratch disease node?	Drain it
In cases of severe cat scratch disease or immunocompromise, how should it be treated?	Azithromycin or Bactrim® first choice – IV or IM gentamicin also used
How long will it take for all symptoms of cat scratch disease to disappear?	Weeks to months (nodes resolve last)
Unilateral proptosis, lid swelling, and fever could be signs of what dangerous syndrome?	**Cavernous sinus syndrome (infectious etiology)**
What infections put patients at special risk for developing cavernous sinus syndrome?	***Any* facial infection (including dental, sinus, & significant acne)**

How great is the mortality from infectious cavernous sinus syndrome?	About 25 %
How useful are blood cultures for treatment of infectious cavernous sinus syndrome?	Actually quite useful – 70 % will grow something
How long should you treat infectious cavernous sinus syndrome?	**Approximately 4 weeks *after* symptoms resolve**
What unfortunate surprise often occurs with infectious cavernous sinus syndrome?	Relapse (locally) or development of embolic abscesses about 4 weeks *after treatment is completed*
What is the usual long-term outcome for patients who <u>recover</u> from infectious cavernous sinus syndrome?	Long-term cranial nerve defects
If infectious cavernous sinus syndrome is not rapidly treated, how will it present?	Meningitis/overwhelming sepsis
What is the main physical finding to look for with a case of cellulitis (suggests you might want to admit the person)?	**Lymphangitis** **(aka lymphangitic spread)**
Facial cellulitis due to what organism often leads to pneumonia, arthritis/ osteomyelitis, and other disseminated foci of infection?	Haemophilus influenza type B
Patients suspected of having cavernous sinus syndrome should have what radiological study?	**MRI with & without gadolinium** (CT is okay but not the gold standard)
Cervical motion tenderness on gyn exam indicates what general problem?	**Peritonitis** (may or may not be gyn related)
What do we use KOH preps to identify, in a gyn patient?	**Yeast (Candida) infection**
What is the trouble with treating vaginal yeast infections with the one-time dose of fluconazole?	**1. Costs the same as other regimens** **2. <u>No</u> symptom relief for at least 1–2 days**

(2)

For any patient found to have cervicitis, what two infections *must* you presumptively treat?

Chlamydia & gonorrhea

What is the most cost-effective treatment regimen for gonorrheal/chlamydial cervicitis?

Ceftriaxone 250 mg IM or Cefixime 400 mg PO

+

Doxycycline, 100 mg PO BID × 7 days

What is the problem with treating adolescents with the doxycycline STD regimen?

(4)

1. **Poor compliance due to BID dosing**
2. **7 days of treatment**
3. **Need to fill prescription**
4. **High stakes for future fertility**

What treatment regimen for gonorrhea/chlamydial cervicitis can you give *during your patient's visit* to ensure compliance?

Ceftriaxone 250 mg IM × 1

+

Azithromycin 1 g PO × 1
(can also give single PO dose of 2 g azithromycin alone, but nasty lower GI side effects usually follow)

Gram-negative diplococci seen with cervicitis = what infection?

Gonorrhea

What exam <u>must</u> be performed in females presenting with cervicitis or vaginal yeast infections?

A bimanual pelvic exam

Should a patient with cervicitis have any pain, or other abnormal findings, on gyn exam?

**No –
Anything else suggests PID, ectopic pregnancy, etc.**

How is the ulcer of chancroid different from the initial syphilitic ulcer (which is also called a chancre)?

The syphilis ulcer is <u>painless</u>

How are the ulcers of chancroid different from those seen in HSV?

Chancroid ulcers are <u>deep</u> with undermined edges

(HSV ulcers are very shallow, <u>not</u> undermined, & multiple)

Like HSV, chancroid requires what condition to infect a person?

A break in the skin (including an abrasion)

What microbe causes chancroid?	**Haemophilus ducreyi** (*Gram negative*)
Under what circumstances is chancroid transmitted?	**Sexual contact with someone with an ulcer**
What three other STDs should be considered in individuals who have developed chancroid?	**10 % coinfection with HSV, syphilis, or HIV** (all also transmitted via breaks in skin)
How is chancroid treated?	**Azithromycin** **1 g PO × 1** **Or** **Ceftriaxone** **250 mg IM × 1** (Cipro 3 days & E-mycin 7 days are also options)
Regional lymphadenopathy usually accompanies chancroid. What complication can this lead to?	**Fluctuant or draining bubo** (A bubo is an inflamed lymph node)
How is chancroid diagnosed?	**Clinically** (a follow-up culture to confirm is the gold standard)
What three chlamydial bacteria affect humans?	1. *C. trachomatis* 2. *C. pneumoniae* 3. *C. psittaci*
Which type of chlamydia is usually responsible for chlamydial pneumonia *in infants*?	*Chlamydia trachomatis*
Which type of chlamydia is responsible for conjunctival infection & blindness in the developing world?	*C. trachomatis*
Which type of chlamydia is the common STD?	*C. trachomatis*
Which chlamydial type is usually responsible for chlamydial pneumonia in adults & older children?	*C. pneumoniae*

Chlamydial pneumonia causes approximately what proportion of childhood community-acquired pneumonias (CAP)?	20–25 %
How do most patients with chlamydial pneumonia present?	<u>Asymptomatic</u> – they don't present
How do infants generally acquire chlamydial pneumonia?	Via vaginal delivery (although C/S does not fully prevent it)
How is *Chlamydia psittaci* acquired?	Inhaled bird excrement or bird secretions (The bird may be healthy or sick)
In addition to chlamydial pneumonia, what other problems can *Chlamydia psittaci* sometimes cause?	Bronchitis, pharyngitis, & otitis media (nasal discharge is common with all 3)
What is the buzzword for chlamydial infection on microscopic evaluation?	Inclusion bodies (It's an obligatory <u>intracellular</u> bacteria)
How is *Chlamydia pneumoniae* acquired?	Inhaled aerosolized droplets
Do infants with *C. trachomatis* have a fever?	**No**
Do children with *C. pneumoniae* have a fever?	**Generally <u>yes</u>**
In general, how are chlamydial infections treated?	Macrolides
What is the overall probability of resistance to erythromycin in chlamydial infection?	20 %
In a case of known maternal GU chlamydial infection, is treatment with topical erythromycin to the conjunctivae sufficient?	**No – it will not eliminate nasopharyngeal colonization**

If you suspect chlamydial infection, but the immunofluorescent study for Chlamydia is negative, what does this mean?

Nothing

(>50 % of chlamydial infections have negative results)

If a mother with untreated GU chlamydial infection delivers a baby, how should you treat the (asymptomatic) infant?

You don't – monitor for signs of infection

If a mother delivers a baby who develops a chlamydial infection, what is the appropriate treatment?

Oral erythromycin × 14 days

(don't forget that mom and partner(s) need treatment as well)

After completion of an antibiotic course for neonatal chlamydia infection, what should be done?

**Follow-up –
Erythromycin is only 80 % effective in eradicating chlamydial infections, so a second course could be needed**

What are the typical CXR findings of chlamydial pneumonia (infants)?

- **Bilateral infiltrates**
- **Hyperinflation**

If an infant is found to have chlamydial infection, what else must you do, in addition to treating the chlamydia?

Look for other STDs

(syphilis, Hep B, HIV, gonorrhea, etc.)

Although humoral immunity is important in preventing and fighting varicella virus (antibodies), what immune component is most critical to preventing severe disease?

Cell-mediated immunity
(T-cell system)

What organ systems may be affected by varicella zoster, if it disseminates?

Basically, any (pneumonitis is especially common)

What is the main effect of congenital varicella infection?

Limb scarring and atrophy

(CNS & eyes may also be affected)

Can a person with herpes zoster (shingles) spread the virus?

**Yes –
Through contact with affected skin;** respiratory transmission is a <u>remote</u> possibility

The severe complications that cause death from varicella infection are more common in adults than children. How much more common?	**35 times!**
How likely are you to catch varicella if you are exposed and are <u>not</u> immune?	98 % (!) (figures vary)
If an individual has had chicken pox, is he or she immune for life?	Generally yes (reinfection is possible, but it is usually mild)
What patient groups are at highest risk for varicella complications? (6) (two age groups) (one medication) (four conditions)	1. Infants *3 months* – 1 year 2. Adolescents/adults 3. Chronic aspirin therapy 4. Immunocompromised 5. Pulmonary disease (incl. asthma) 6. Pregnant women 7. Chronic skin disorders (severe eczema, etc.)
In what order does the varicella rash develop? **(4)**	1. **Macule** 2. **Papule** 3. **Vesicle** 4. **Crust**
In addition to the typical rash stages, what other buzzwords describe the varicella rash? **(2)**	1. **Rash in various stages over body** 2. **"Dewdrop on a rose petal" appearance**
What are the typical seasons for varicella?	Winter & spring
Is it alright to use aspirin or NSAIDs for children with chicken pox?	No – Aspirin + varicella = Reye's syndrome NSAIDS + varicella = increased incidence of bacterial superinfection
When should antiviral therapy be given to chicken pox patients? **(1 situation)** **(2 age groups)** **(4 medical conditions)**	1. **Hospitalized patients** 2. **Newborns & adolescents** 3. **Immunocompromised** (*incl. those on inhaled steroids*) 4. **Chronic skin or lung disease** 5. **Pregnant**

What type of isolation is needed for hospitalized varicella patients?

Contact and respiratory (while vesicles present)

How long should an exposed, varicella susceptible individual be isolated? (if hospitalized)

From days 8–21 *after rash develops in the index case*

Who usually has more severe disease, the index case, or the secondary cases, in varicella infections?

Secondary cases, in general

In current practice, which patient groups should <u>not</u> receive varicella vaccine?

(3)

1. **Infants <1 year**
2. **Immunocompromised (but some HIV+ should get it)**
3. **Pregnant women**
4. **Patients with malignancies of the blood/bone marrow or lymphatic system**
5. **Recently received blood products (up to 11 months prior)**

What is required for maximum protection from the varicella vaccine?

A second dose (the regimen is now two doses, to minimize declining immunity after vaccination)

If a varicella non-immune patient is exposed to varicella, but cannot receive the vaccine, what other prevention strategy should be considered?

VZ-IG

During what portion of pregnancy can varicella cause birth defects?

Between the 8th and 20th weeks

Teratogenic varicella affects what portion(s) of the developing embryo/fetus?

The ectoderm (eyes, skin, CNS, & limbs are affected)

Why are the limbs affected in teratogenic varicella?

Damage to the ectodermal structures of the brachial & lumbar nerve plexi causes limb abnormalities

How should you care for a pregnant mother exposed to varicella in the first or the second trimester?

VZ-IG if not immune –
Acyclovir if chicken pox has already developed

If the embryo or the fetus is infected by varicella in the 1st or the 2nd trimesters, what is the likely outcome?

Bad –
death or severe CNS damage

Although varicella can have teratogenic effects, <u>congenital</u> varicella means something else. What does it mean?

Maternal infection developed in the last 3 weeks of gestation, or first week after birth

If the infant develops congenital varicella infection, when will his/her illness become clinically apparent?

First 10 days of life

If the mother develops varicella in the last 3 weeks of pregnancy, how likely is the fetus to develop varicella?

Quite likely –
¼ to ½ will contract the disease

What determines the severity of congenital varicella infection (mainly)?

When the mother is infected – <u>≤5 days</u> before delivery is *bad*

(no time for maternal antibody to be made & transferred)

What is the pattern of the rash seen in congenital varicella infection?

<u>Centripetal</u> but sparing extremities

(centripetal = going toward the center of the body)

If the newborn does not have maternal antibodies to varicella, peripartum infection can be quite severe. How does varicella typically cause death?

Due to pulmonary involvement

If a mother develops varicella >5 days prior to delivery, should her infant receive immunoglobulin?

No – the infant is assumed to have already received maternal immunoglobulin

If VZ-IG is given empirically to a neonate, how long must the infant be kept in respiratory isolation?

28 days

(immunoglobulin extends the incubation period)

What is the other name for perleche?   **Angular cheilosis**

What organism is generally responsible for perleche?

Candida
(plus licking corners of mouth, braces, or bad overbite)

In an older child or adult, consider staph aureus infection, iron or riboflavin deficiency

Are infants with thrush consistently symptomatic?

No – some are asymptomatic

A weepy and erythematous rash in skin folds, confluent, with a scaling edge suggests what problem?

Intertriginous candidiasis

How is intertriginous candidiasis treated?

Keep area dry

+

Nystatin cream
(or other topical antifungal)

How is disseminated candidiasis treated?

IV amphotericin B × 6 weeks

OR

Fluconazole (static) & the newer "fungin" drugs (fungicidal)
(*Example: micafungin*)

In settings of either immunocompromise or imbalance of bacteria, oral thrush often progresses to what difficult-to-manage problem?

Esophagitis

Candidal infections regularly cause what secondary problem?
(a general, body-wide problem)

Allergic reactions (rash, itch, asthma, exacerbations, a type of colitis, etc.)

Scattered erythematous papules **in the diaper area, or a confluent rash with a** *scalloped or a scaling* **border = ?**

Diaper dermatitis (candida)

Is nystatin used to treat vaginal candidiasis?

No –
use one of the "azoles"

Which famous fungus comes from the dry soil in the southwestern USA?	Coccidioides
How long is the incubation period for coccidioides?	Up to 30 days
What is the common name for the illness it causes?	San Joaquin Valley fever or Desert Rheumatism (because it often causes joint pain & myalgias)
What is the usual course for a coccidioidomycosis infection?	Asymptomatic pulmonary infections (60 %)
Which ethnic groups are especially likely to have bad episodes of coccidiodomycosis?	Hispanic African American & Filipino Mnemonic: Think of half (HAAF) an infected *coccyx*, having trouble breathing on a trip to the desert to remember this disease, and the ethnic groups it especially affects!
Adults with symptomatic pulmonary coccidioidomycosis complain of hemoptysis. How do children present?	1. Fever, cough, pleuritic chest pain 2. Arthralgia and myalgia 3. Night sweats 4. Maculopapular lower body rash
What finding on micro exam (from any source) suggests coccidioidomycosis?	Large "spherules"
A skin test (delayed-type hypersensitivity) is available to aid in the diagnosis of coccidioidomycosis. In what situation is the test often falsely negative?	Disseminated disease (due to anergy)
How is disseminated coccidioidomycosis treated?	Ampho B, generally
If it is able to disseminate, where does coccidioides like to go?	Bones & joints Lymph nodes CNS Abdominal sites

What causes Condyloma acuminata?

**HPV –
human papillomavirus**
(aka papova viridae)

What is the histologic buzzword for condyloma?

"Koilocytosis"
(& atypical nuclei)

koilocytosis means an empty space near the nucleus

How long can the incubation period for HPV last?

Several years

How common is HPV infection?

Very **common**

(it is the *most common STD* –
at least 20 % of sexually active women are infected)

What easily accessed substance makes it much easier to visualize areas infected with HPV?

Acetic acid
(leave on for 5 min – affected areas turn white)

What is the usual course of HPV infection?

Like herpes, the immune system eventually keeps the virus from manifesting & may eliminate it

Does genital Condyloma acuminata in a child indicate sexual abuse?

Sometimes –
It should always be investigated but close nonsexual contact can also transmit the virus

A vaccine for HPV infection is now available. What is the main restriction on who can get the vaccine?

It is given to patients between the ages of 9 and 26 years old (target age for vaccination is 11–12 years old)

Is HPV vaccination useful for boys, as well as girls?

Yes –
The quadrivalent vaccine prevents infection with strains linked to genital cancers in males

What is the other name for neonatal conjunctivitis?

Ophthalmia neonatorum

Does GC conjunctivitis lead to blindness?

Yes, without prompt therapy

Why must conjunctivitis <u>never</u> be treated with steroid drops by a primary care doctor?	Could accelerate an undiagnosed <u>herpes</u> keratitis
What is the buzzword for herpes keratitis on physical exam?	"Dendritic" (branching) pattern of fluorescein uptake
What is the other name for croup?	**Laryngotracheobronchitis**
What causes croup?	**A variety of viruses** (the symptom constellation defines the disorder rather than the causative agent)
What three symptoms characterize "croup?"	1. **"Barky" cough** 2. **Inspiratory stridor** 3. **Hoarseness**
How is "spasmodic croup" different from regular croup?	1. **It occurs only at night** 2. **Child appears well** (or minimally ill)
During what season is croup most often seen?	Winter
What is the typical age & gender for a croup patient?	**<3 years** (usually 2) **and male**
What is the buzzword for croup on X-ray, and why does it occur?	• **"Steeple sign"** • **Subglottic narrowing due to inflammation near the cricoid**
What diagnostics are useful for croup patients? **(2)**	**Pulse ox** (r/o hypoxia) & **AP & lateral neck X-ray**
In addition to "steeple sign", what else should you be looking for on X-ray if you suspect croup? (3)	1. Foreign body 2. The "thumb" of epiglottitis 3. Retropharyngeal infection or abscess
For croup patients requiring medical intervention, what therapies are useful? **(2)**	1. **Racemic epi** (nebulized) 2. **Steroids** (usually a single dose of dexamethasone – 45 h $T_{1/2}$)

What simple interventions have long been thought to improve symptoms in croup patients, although *recent data* **does not support this?**
(2)

Humidified air

&

Cold air

How long must you observe a patient who requires racemic epi treatment for croup, before discharging to home?

At least 4 h after treatment

(some patients rebound & worsen after treatment)

Recurrent croup suggests that a child may be suffering from one of the two underlying disorders. What are they?

1. **Subglottic stenosis/congenital anomaly**
2. **GE reflux**

Cryptococcus usually affects what organ system?

CNS
(occasionally lungs & other areas)

How is cryptococcal meningitis treated?

Amphotericin B

+

Flucytosine
(6 weeks)

Recurrence of cryptococcal meningitis is common. How do we prevent this in the immunocompromised?

Maintenance fluconazole

What is the prognosis for cryptococcal meningitis (properly treated)?

Very good

(*Fatal without treatment, by the way*)

What special CSF tests should be done if cryptococcal meningitis is suspected?
(2)

India ink stain

&

Cryptococcal antigen

Where is *Cryptococcus neoformans* found in nature?

Pigeon droppings & soil

Are immunocompromised hosts at risk for cryptococcal recurrences?

Yes
(at least 1 year of regular follow-up is required)

What are the two common presentations of pulmonary cryptococcosis?

Asymptomatic

&

Cough & hemoptysis

What are the symptoms of cutaneous larva migrans?	*Itching* & serpiginous erythematous lines (serpiginous = snakelike)
What usually causes cutaneous larva migrans?	Hookworms in the wrong host
What is the incubation period for cutaneous larva migrans?	7–10 days
What disease related to cutaneous larva migrans develops after swimming in filariaform-infested waters?	Swimmer's itch
How is cutaneous larva migrans treated?	Topical or oral thiabendazole (will spontaneously resolve but is very annoying to the patient)
Two types of bacteria cause the clinical illness known as Ehrlichiosis. Which two bacteria are they?	Anaplasma phagocytophilum & *Ehrlichia chaffeensis* (*Both gram-negative intracellular coccobacilli*)
What makes the two Ehrlichia bacterial species so unusual?	They live within the phagosomes of immune cells
Which TWO types of immune cells are affected in Ehrlichiosis?	Granulocytes with Anaplasma infection & Monocytes with *E. chaffeensis* infection
Anaplasmosis is an alternative name for which disorder?	Ehrlichiosis due to Anaplasma – It is also known as human granulocytic anaplasmosis (HGA)
The vector & geographic distribution of disease are the same for Lyme disease & which form of Ehrlichiosis?	Anaplasma phagocytophilum Ehrlichiosis
Geographically, where does the other form of Ehrlichiosis mainly occur?	Southeast, South central, & Midatlantic USA – Lone Star tick vector (*Amblyomma americanum*)

What makes the two Ehrlichia bacterial species so unusual?

They live within the phagosomes of immune cells

(Gram-negative, intracellular coccobacilli)

What unusual micro finding is reported after about a week of Ehrlichiosis infection?

Intracellular inclusions in a mulberry or a morula shape – it is lots of tiny bacteria multiplying in the cell!

Diagnostic for Ehrlichiosis!!!

How is Ehrlichiosis acquired?

Tick bite

(In the USA – mainly Ixodes scapularis & pacificus for Anaplasma, Amblyomma for E. chaffeensis)

Is Ehrlichiosis seen outside the USA?

Yes –
The Anaplasma type is seen in Europe & Asia & other species cause Ehrlichiosis elsewhere

What lab abnormalities do you expect to see in the CBC of an Ehrlichiosis patient?
(3)

1. Leukopenia
2. Thrombocytopenia
3. +/− anemia

What non-CBC lab abnormalities are expected in Ehrlichiosis?
(2)

↑ LFTs (usually ALT)

&

Hyponatremia

What is the drug of choice for Ehrlichiosis?

Doxycycline
(at least 7 days – alternative is chloramphenicol)

What other infectious disease sometimes co-occurs with Ehrlichiosis?

Lyme disease
(titers should be sent)

What is the most common chief complaint in children presenting with Ehrlichiosis?

Bad headache

Which patients are at special risk for more severe Ehrlichiosis?

Asplenic & immunocompromised patients

(RMSF-type presentation)

Where does CMV hide when it is in a latent stage?

Peripheral monocytes

What is the hallmark of CMV infection on microscopic exam?
(2)

Very large cells

&

Intranuclear **inclusion bodies**

In utero CMV infection is the most common cause of which congenital problem?

Congenital deafness

Which body systems can CMV affect – especially in the immunocompromised?

Essentially all of them

What medication may be used to treat CMV?

Ganciclovir

(Foscarnet is second line currently)

Which medication is currently the mainstay for CMV prevention in transplant patients, & in treating CMV retinitis?

Valganciclovir

What effect do CMV medications have on the virus?

They are static only

How common is it for asymptomatic individuals to shed CMV in body secretions?

Very common

In the USA, approximately how common is CMV exposure?

Approximately 50 % of the population

(these individuals often continue to shed the virus)

What is the main problem caused by cryptosporidiosis?

Secretory diarrhea

What is cryptosporidiosis?

A protozoan spread via fecal-oral contamination (human or animal)

Which patients have the greatest difficulty with cryptosporidial infection?

Immunocompromised

&

Kids <5 years

Although there is no entirely effective treatment for cryptosporidiosis, which medication is considered to be the drug of choice?

Nitazoxanide

(used with immunocompromised patients)

(*Paromomycin +/– azithromycin is still sometimes used, but is less effective than nitazoxanide*)

What unusual source is sometimes the vector of infection for cryptosporidiosis?

Apple cider

(unless it is pasteurized – crypto lives well in apple cider for a month!)

(Remember that EHEC is in apple *juice*)

How can public or private water supplies be protected from cryptosporidial contamination?

Filtration systems

How is cryptosporidiosis definitively diagnosed?

Oocysts in stool

(often hard to find, must send 3 specimens from 3 different days, minimum)

Which viral group most commonly causes hand–foot–mouth disease?

Coxsackie viruses

What feature of hand–foot–mouth causes the biggest problem?

"Vesiculoulcerative" stomatitis – may produce dehydration

What is the usual pattern for development of hand–foot–mouth diseases?

Oral ulcers,

then,

Papular or vesicular exanthem on hands/feet (non-tender, non-pruritic)

Although lidocaine (viscous) is sometimes given with other ingredients as a mouthwash to relieve oral pain, why can this be a dangerous practice?

Direct absorption from mucous membranes skips the "first pass" effect & can deliver a fairly sizable lido dose (→*arrhythmias*)

Which two viruses typically cause a macular rash on the palms & soles? (unusual pattern!)

Echovirus 16 (Boston exanthem)

&

Coxsackie virus

Where, specifically, does herpes hide when it's latent (not active)?

Sensory neural ganglia (hence the paresthesias that often precede an outbreak when it starts "creeping out")

Does neonatal HSV infection require contact with a herpes lesion to develop?

No!
(only 25 % of mothers with affected infants have a history of or current infection with HSV, and some c/s infants still develop HSV)

Will a patient with herpes encephalitis have skin or mucous membrane/oral lesions?	No
Does c-section delivery prevent transmission of herpes to the neonate?	No (although it is still standard of care if lesions are present)
What is the buzzword for herpes infection on micro preparation?	Multinucleated giant cells
How is HSV encephalitis definitively diagnosed?	Brain biopsy or PCR of CSF
What will the CSF profile of a patient with herpes encephalitis usually look like?	1. WBC pleocytosis – <u>mainly lymphs</u> 2. High protein 3. High RBCs (even without trauma, due to hemorrhagic necrosis)
Are CSF viral cultures for HSV useful?	Usually not – Often negative even with clear HSV infection
What is the preferred imaging study for suspected HSV encephalitis?	MRI
How are serious herpex simplex infections treated?	IV acyclovir for 21 days (vidarabine is sometimes added for encephalitis)
Medical professionals are at risk for herpes in unusual locations if they fail to use universal precautions. What is the most common site for the "occupationally exposed" to have a lesion?	**Fingertip – aka "Herpetic Whitlow"**
What sport is associated with herpes outbreaks on unusual portions of the body?	**Wrestling – They have many abrasions & pick it up from the mat**
What is the most common complication of long courses of acyclovir in young children?	**Neutropenia** (25 % with 6 months of use)

Where does Hantavirus come from in nature?	Rodents
How do humans become infected with Hantavirus?	Inhalation of dried excretions/secretions
What age groups are most commonly affected by Hanta pulmonary syndrome, & Hanta infection generally?	Children & healthy young adults
Are the rodents that carry Hantavirus ill appearing?	No – they have a chronic infection
What are the main clinical features of Hanta pulmonary syndrome? (2)	1. Respiratory failure (alveoli fill with protein-rich fluid) 2. Cardiac depression (low cardiac output with high vascular resistance)
What are the typical activities associated with catching Hanta infection?	Sweeping, cleaning, or construction in a rodent-infested building
What symptoms often occur in the early stages of Hanta infection?	• Fever • Myalgia & headache • GI distress (n/v/d & pain)
Is cough common in the early stages of Hanta infection?	*No* – it comes just before the very serious phase (*pulmonary edema and cardiac suppression*)
Will you see an enlarged cardiac silhouette in Hanta pulmonary syndrome?	No – The CXR looks like CHF, but this is due to profound leakiness mainly, not cardiac dilation
Which lab values can be a clue to the presence of Hanta, if followed over time? (3)	1. The platelet count (it falls during the prodrome) 2. Immature WBC forms are seen in the peripheral blood 3. IgM to Hanta will be present
Can Hantavirus spread from person to person?	Generally, no (one S. American type can, but it is not likely to be on the boards)

If patients survive the shock phase of Hanta pulmonary syndrome, what is the usual prognosis?

Good
(some residual pulmonary problems may persist but they are mild)

What is the usual cause of impetigo?

Staph aureus

What are the two forms of impetigo?

Bullous

&

Non-bullous
(this one more likely to be caused by other organisms, mainly GABHS, in addition to *S. aureus*)

How does impetigo cause infection?

Bacteria invade the skin at points of minor trauma

In Fitz-Hugh-Curtis syndrome, what is the problem with the right upper quadrant?

Perihepatitis

(infection around the liver capsule, <u>not</u> in the liver itself, usually coming from a gyn source)

"Early" infection with Group B Strep produces what sort of neonatal infection?

Sepsis in the first week of life

What factors, related to the birth itself, make Group B Strep infection more likely?

1. Younger age
2. Lower SES
3. Multiple sex partners
4. History of STDS

If microabscesses are seen on the internal organs of a septic newborn, what is the likely cause of the sepsis?

Listeria monocytogenes

If the mother of a septic newborn has had "flu-like symptoms," what is the likely cause of the infant's sepsis?

Listeria

If the mother of a septic infant was asymptomatic during pregnancy/delivery, what is the likely cause of the infant's sepsis?

Group B strep

(don't forget *N. meningitis* is also a possibility)

In adolescents, how is PID usually treated?

Inpatient, due to risk to fertility if compliance is poor

(usually gentamicin + clindamycin – both meds have "mice" in the name)

Outpatient treatment is also acceptable, if the adolescent meets criteria for outpatient treatment, including likelihood of compliance

How does an osteomyelitis from pseudomonas get started?

Classically, the vignette will be a nail through a sneaker (rubber sole)

Which other patient groups are likely to develop pseudomonal infections?

1. **Burn patients**
2. **Mechanically ventilated (waterborne)**
3. **CF**
4. **Leukemia**

In otherwise healthy folks, what pseudomonal infection is fairly common?

Otitis externa

Which cephalosporin is frequently used against pseudomonas?

Ceftazidime

A child who becomes sick while staying on a dairy farm (fevers, myalgia) may have what dairy-related disorder?

Brucellosis
Mnemonic:
Picture a cow saying "BRUUUCE" instead of "MOOO!"

An STD + arthritis or multiple skin nodules = what diagnosis?

Gonorrhea

Arthritis + right *upper* quadrant tenderness in a female = what diagnosis?

Gonorrhea – specifically Fitz-Hugh-Curtis syndrome

Since botulism is caused by a bacterium, why don't we treat it with antibiotics?
(3 reasons)

1. The toxin is the problem, not the bacteria
2. Killing the spores may result in *increased* toxin release in the gut (infant botulism)
3. Some antibiotics actually make the effects of the toxin worse

How does botulism cause problems?	**It blocks <u>release</u> of Ach**
If you give the "tensilon test" to a botulism patient, will it be positive?	**No –** **it is positive in myasthenia gravis** (tensilon inhibits acetylcholinesterase, but that doesn't help if there's no ACh)
How does botulism cause problems for children & adults?	**Preformed toxin is ingested** (usually from canned goods)
How is infant botulism different from the disorder seen in children and adults?	*Spores* **are ingested, these grow in the gut,** *then* **release toxin** (Doesn't happen in older children, because gut flora prevent significant growth by the botulinum spores)
An infant with poor feeding, ptosis, and/or descending paralysis most likely has what disorder?	**Botulism** (even if honey ingestion is <u>not</u> mentioned)
If an infant's mother has a history of syphilis – properly treated – does the newborn infant require treatment?	**No –** **but IgG titers should be followed & they should fall over time if the antibodies came from the mom**
If a mother is being treated with penicillin for syphilis, will her in utero fetus be treated at the same time?	**Yes –** <u>**PCN**</u> **crosses the** <u>**placenta**</u>**!**
A newborn with a maculopapular rash, hepatosplenomegaly, and "peeling skin," is likely to have what disorder?	**Syphilis**
Which test is more specific and reliable when you are looking for possible syphilis – VDRL or FTA-Abs?	**FTA-Abs** – (fluorescent treponemal antigen antibodies – this test remains positive for life)
If a patient sustains a "dirty wound," how do you know whether a tetanus booster is needed?	If it is <u>more than 5 years</u> from the child's most recent booster (or original immunization) a booster is needed

In addition to obviously dirty wounds, what three other important categories of wounds are considered to be dirty?

1. **Crush injuries**
2. **Burns**
3. **Frostbite**

If a child has a "clean" wound, how do you know whether a tetanus booster is required?

>10 years since last immunization

What bacterium is especially associated with hemolytic uremic syndrome (HUS)?

E. coli
(especially *0157:H7*)

Vignettes in which the child has consumed spoiled milk or undercooked beef are likely to involve what bacterium?

E. coli

(Think of that unfortunate fast food incident a few years back . . . in which several children died due to contaminated burgers!)

What is one simple way to differentiate staph scalded skin syndrome from the erythema multiforme group of disorders?

Staph scalded skin should *not* involve the mucosa

What is toxic epidermal necrolysis (TEN) caused by?

Hypersensitivity reaction (not a toxin) – **usually it's a reaction to medication**

What causes staph scalded skin syndrome?

Exotoxin **from particular Staph bacteria**

What causes toxic shock syndrome?

Toxin-producing Staph (occasionally strep can do it also)

If you are treating a patient for Strep who is PCN allergic, what other medication can you use?

Clindamycin

What is the drug of choice for tularemia?

Streptomycin

(Gentamicin is an acceptable alternative)

How is tularemia acquired on the boards?
(& how is it acquired in real life?)

Boards – involvement with rabbit meat or skinning

(real life – mainly tick-borne)

Burn patients are especially at risk for what *fungal* infection?

Candidiasis

Burn patients are especially at risk for what *bacterial* infection?

Pseudomonas

Patients on TPN are especially likely to develop what fungal infection?

Candidiasis

What virus likes to cause viral meningitis during the summer months?

Enterovirus
(also causes rash & high fever)

If a child has a swollen parotid gland, but is fully immunized, what causes should you think of?
(4)

1. **Obstructing stone**
2. **Bacterial infection** (toxic appearance)
3. **Viral infection**
4. **Bulimia, if it's bilateral**

If a child has not completed his or her immunizations, or has come to the country from abroad, and has swollen parotid glands, what disease should you consider?

Mumps

What is the "formal name" for roseola? (it's often listed this way in answer choices)

HHV-6
(Human herpesvirus type 6)

What is the typical pattern seen in roseola infection (usual clinical course)?

1. **3–5 days' high fever**
2. **Maculopapular rash when the fever ends**
3. **Complete recovery**

What is the formal name for the type of measles associated with birth defects?

Rubella – also known as German measles

Mnemonic:
Imagine an infant speaking German wearing a "bell" that hangs over her heart. The bell is to warn others when she's coming, because she often bumps into things, due to poor vision (cataracts)

If a pregnant mother is found to be measles (rubella) non-immune, should you give the vaccine?

No – it is a live vaccine & can cause problems itself

What two defects are seen most commonly in infants affected by rubella?	PDA (& other heart issues) & Cataracts
Regular measles (rubeola) has an average incubation period of one to one-and-a-half weeks. When are patients most likely to be contagious?	**5 days <u>before</u> until 5 days <u>after</u> the rash first appears**
In what age group is measles (rubeola) most often seen?	Preschool
How is rubeola spread?	**Contact with secretions** **&** **Aerosolized droplets inhaled**
Is measles (rubeola) seen in native-born US children?	**Yes**
What are the buzzwords for the classic measles (rubeola) presentation? **(5)**	**Fever** **Cough** **Coryza** **Conjunctivitis** **Cutaneous rash** **(+/– Koplik spots in the mouth)**
Should HIV patients receive the MMR (live) vaccine?	**<u>Yes</u> – the risk of the diseases is worse than the risk of the immunization**
If an infant is exposed to rubeola, what should be done? **(2 steps)**	**1. Give MMR within 3 days of exposure** (Mnemonic: 3 letters in MMR means you have 3 days) **2. Give immunoglobulin within 6 days of exposure**
If an infant has received rubeola immunoglobulin, does that change the protocol for MMR vaccination?	**Yes – in addition to the initial vaccine, another dose should be given in 5 months**
If a child receives the MMR before he or she is 1 year old, is reimmunization needed?	*Yes –* **when the child is more than 1 year old**

In addition to supportive care, what specific intervention is recommended for a child with measles by WHO, regardless of the country of origin?	Vitamin A (one dose on two consecutive days, to reduce possible complications)
If a child has a known exposure to a bat, but there was no bite or other contact, is any intervention needed?	Generally, *yes* – Especially if the exposure was in an enclosed space – Immunize & give IgG for rabies
Do rodents carry rabies?	No – Do not immunize for squirrel bites, etc.
Which animals are *most likely* to carry rabies in North America?	Bats, fox, skunks, raccoons (local patterns vary)
If the patient was bitten by a domestic animal, should rabies prevention treatment be started?	No, if 1. the animal has proof of immunization or 2. the animal can be observed for signs of illness for 10 days, and 3. the bite was *not* to the head (a bite on the head would require treatment, even if the animal is being observed)
If a child is bitten by a possibly rabid animal, how should the child be treated?	1. Human rabies immunoglobulin is injected at the site of the bite 2. Series of **4** rabies vaccinations should be started (note that this is a CHANGE from the previous 5) 3. Wash & debride wound
Why are unprovoked animal bites more worrisome for rabies, than those that occur when the patient was interacting with the animal?	Unprovoked = higher probability the animal is rabid
Why are bites that occurred in areas closer to the brain more likely to cause problems, in terms of rabies?	The virus migrates along the nerves to the brain – the shorter the distance, the faster it arrives!
Is rabies common in animals in other parts of the world?	YES – very common!

Are travelers at increased risk for rabies, if they are not specifically working with animals?

YES – dogs are the most common source for rabies amongst travelers & contact with animals in public areas is enough to contract the disease!

If a patient returns after a trip, and was bitten by a dog but didn't receive rabies prophylaxis, should you still give it?

YES –
The incubation can sometimes last a long time, and even partial immunization increases chances of survival

If your patient contracts rabies, can it be treated?

Not really –
There are some experimental protocols, but it is essentially 100 % fatal

What is the histopathological "buzzword" for rabies infection in the CNS?

"Negri bodies" are seen – dark inclusions in brain neurons

Seizure in the first 4 weeks of life, especially if it involves the temporal lobe or the CSF has no organisms on Gram stain, should make you consider what organism?

HSV

Is it safe for HIV-infected moms to breastfeed?

No – in developed countries, the risks outweigh the benefits

What is the most common deep infection of the head and neck, and which age group tends to get it?

**Peritonsillar abscess –
Young adults & adolescents**

Aside from the patient's discomfort, what is the most concerning aspect of a peritonsillar abscess?

**Spread to the adjacent tissue planes producing
1. serious infection &
2. airway compromise**

What is the most common organism found in *retropharyngeal* abscesses?

β-Hemolytic strep

At what age does retropharyngeal abscess typically occur?

6 months to 3 years

How does retropharyngeal abscess present?	**Fever** **Ill to toxic appearing** **Stridor** **Dysphagia** **+/− Drooling** **Refusal to eat** **Little movement (it hurts)**
What is the most feared complication of lateral pharyngeal space infections?	**Septic thrombophlebitis of the jugular vein** (***Lemierre's syndrome***)
What is the usual bacterial agent in Lemierre's syndrome?	**Fusobacterium** **(others are possible, and is often polymicrobial)**
A teenager presents with a sore throat, but seems genuinely ill, with fever & rigors. What serious disorder should you consider?	**Lemierre's syndrome** (*admit − IV antibiotics!*)
If a child develops pneumonia following an episode of the flu, what is the likely organism?	**Staph aureus**
Would oral Augmentin® (amoxicillin/ clavulanate) be an acceptable way to treat staph aureus pneumonia?	Usually
When is it not alright to treat staph aureus with oral Augmentin®?	If the patient is bacteremic (or otherwise very ill − or allergic, of course)
What are the most likely organisms for CNS shunt infections? (2)	Staph aureus & Staph epidermidis
Osteomyelitis, on the peds boards, will normally be caused by what organism?	Staph aureus
Osteomyelitis that follows stepping on a nail, after it goes through your tennis shoe, will give you what type of osteomyelitis on the boards?	Pseudomonas

Patients with sickle cell disease are more likely than average (& *very* likely on the boards) to develop osteomyelitis due to what organism?	Salmonella
Children with cyanotic congenital heart disease are at increased risk for what very unusual ID problem?	Brain abscess
What is the typical organism seen with the abscesses of congenital heart disease patients?	Staph aureus brain abscesses
What is the drug of choice for MRSA bacteremia?	Vancomycin
Staph aureus is well known for causing what three skin disorders?	1. Impetigo 2. Toxic shock syndrome 3. Staph epidermal necrolysis
Bacteremia in an IV drug abuser or dialysis patient will be due to what organism, on the boards?	Staph aureus
Shock + rash on the boards usually =	**Toxic shock syndrome**
If you see MRSA in outpatients (such as from a furuncle or carbuncle), how should you treat it?	**Clindamycin or Bactrim®**
If you have an MRSA + infection in an outpatient who is also blood culture + for MRSA, how should you treat it?	**<u>IV vancomycin</u>**
If a device has recently been implanted in a patient who later develops toxic shock syndrome, what are the two main actions that must be taken?	<u>Remove</u> the device & Start antibiotics
In addition to Staph aureus, what other organism is especially associated with toxic shock syndrome?	Strep pyogenes

If a patient develops toxic shock syndrome, and has a positive blood culture, what is the organism?	**Staph aureus**
If a patient develops toxic shock syndrome, and blood cultures are negative, what is the organism?	**Strep pyogenes**
Is it alright to treat a staph species with vancomycin if it is sensitive to β-lactams?	No! (too expensive, often less effective in these bugs, & it risks creating vanc-resistant bugs for no reason)
What organism is the most common cause of catheter-related bacteremia?	Staph epidermidis
What organism is the most common cause of bacteremia in patients who have had medical devices implanted?	Staph epi (epidermidis)
How is Staph epidermidis treated?	Vancomycin or a β-lactam, if sensitive
Are there any special situations when you should consider giving <u>more</u> than "just" vancomycin for a methicillin-resistant staph strain?	Yes – May add gentamicin or rifampin for endocarditis Rifampin alone may be added in cases of CNS or osteomyelitis infection
What is the only case in which you should automatically add both rifampin & gentamicin to vancomycin, to treat MRSA/E?	Endocarditis involving a prosthetic valve
Which other medication is generally acceptable to use for MRSA/E, in place of vancomycin?	Daptomycin (lower dose for kids <12 years old)
If no intravascular or bactermia-type illness is suspected, what alternative drugs may be used to treat methicillin-resistant staph species?	Clindamycin & Linezolid
Can Staph epidermidis ever be safely considered a contaminant?	Yes – well-appearing child and one culture bottle positive *only*

What does the rash of toxic shock syndrome look like?	Sunburn – Light red all over, then it peels (desquamates)
What unusual parts of the body are involved in the desquamating rash of TSS?	Palms & soles
If a NICU baby has one culture bottle positive for Staph epi, and the other bottle is negative, is it alright to consider it a contaminant?	No (NICU babies are too unpredictable)

How should you treat Strep pneumo meningitis – initially, before the cultures come back?
(*Popular test item!*)

Vancomycin

+

3rd-generation cephalosporin

If a sensitivity for Strep pneumo comes back saying that it has "intermediate resistance" to PCN, how should you treat the infection?	3rd-generation cephalosporin

If sensitivities on Strep pneumo come back as "highly resistant" to PCN, how should you treat the infection?

Vancomycin

+

3rd-generation cephalosporin

Why is Strep pneumo such an important bug?	It is the most common bacterial cause of most of the important peds infectious diseases (OM, pneumonia, meningitis, bacteremia)
Which kids are most likely to be harboring resistant strep pneumo *in their ears*? (4 factors)	1. Recent antibiotic use 2. Recurrent OM 3. Daycare kids 4. <2 years old

If a child is likely to have resistant OM, what should you treat him or her with?

80–90 mg/kg/day amoxicillin

In an occult bacteremia case, if a blood culture comes back positive for Strep pneumo, what should you do?	Call to check on the child – if sick, call in Abx, if not sick, <u>do nothing</u>

Now that the pentavalent pneumococcal vaccine is routinely administered, how common is the dreaded Strep pneumo bacteremia?

Very uncommon (approximately 0.3 % of febrile children meeting the rule-out bacteremia criteria)

On the boards, how do you diagnose a child with exudative tonsils as having strep throat?

Rapid strep

+

throat culture (if the rapid strep was negative)

When is pharyngitis not likely to be due to strep infection, just based on clinical findings?

If there is cough, rhinorrhea, or other URI symptoms

If a throat culture comes back positive for strep after the rapid strep was negative, should you have the child come in for a follow-up visit?

No –
just call in Abx after notifying the caregiver

What kind of strep normally causes strep pharyngitis?

Strep pyogenes
(Grp A strep)

In infants with pharyngeal group A Strep, what are the symptoms?
(4)

1. Thick, purulent nasal discharge
2. Low-grade fever
3. Decreased feeding
4. Vomiting/abdominal pain

Should infants routinely be checked for group A Strep infection, if they have some matching symptoms?

No –
<18 months should be tested only if there is a Strep-positive contact

(*positive test due to colonization without disease is also possible*)

What is scarlet fever?

Strep throat with a rash (yes, that's all it is)

Why do some patients get a rash with strep throat, & others do not?

It comes from an exotoxin, & only certain streps make it

What do you need to know about the appearance of the scarlet fever rash?
(3 main things)

1. Feels like "sandpaper"
2. Prominent in flexor skin creases
3. "Pastia's Lines" are pathognomonic (lines of erythema in flexor creases)

How is erysipelas different from other staph/strep skin infections?

1. It is tender
2. Usually systemically ill
3. All skin layers & underlying tissues are involved
4. Deep red with a sharp margin

On the boards, how might you want to culture for the Strep pyogenes that causes erysipelas?

"Leading edge culture"
(use a syringe to inject a little saline into the skin of the leading edge, pull back, & culture)

Which type of Strep pyogenes skin infection requires surgical debridement?

Necrotizing fasciitis
("flesh-eating bacteria")

What is the treatment for necrotizing fasciitis?
(2 components)

1. *Surgical debridement*
2. Antibiotics
(PCN and clinda IV, sometimes additional antibiotics until susceptibility is determined)

What treatment for necrotizing fasciitis shows promise, but remains controversial?

Hyperbaric oxygen

IVIG is sometimes with which type of necrotizing fasciitis?

Streptococcal toxic shock syndrome

(less useful in children than adults, though, due to lesser mortality in children)

A child with shock and a rash, but no petechiae has what disorder?

Toxic shock syndrome

True or False – rheumatic fever can *only* develop from pharyngeal group A Strep?

True

Should all Strep pharyngitis be treated with antibiotics?

Yes –
to shorten the course & prevent rheumatic fever

Do all types of Strep pharyngitis have the potential to cause rheumatic fever?

No – only group A Strep can do it

Does antibiotic treatment of group A Strep prevent post-strep glomerulonephritis from happening?

No (not even a little bit)

Can post-strep glomerulonephritis develop after a skin infection with GAS, or only after pharyngitis?

Either one!

What is the other name for group B Strep?

Strep agalactiae
(galacto means milk and "B" stands for bovine cow)

Why is the heart affected in rheumatic fever?

"M" proteins of certain Strep bacteria generate a strong antibody response – and those antibodies are cross-reactive against (all sorts of) cardiac tissues

What is REQUIRED for diagnosing rheumatic fever?

Proof of Strep infection
(positive culture, ASO titer, anti-hyaluronidase or anti-deoxyribonuclease B)

What are the *major* (Jones) criteria for rheumatic fever?

CHorea
Arthritis (polyarthritis)
Nodules (subcutaneous)
Carditis
Erythema marginatum

(*Mnemonic*: CHANCE – *You won't have a chance in life without good heart valves!*)

How many major & minor criteria are required to make the rheumatic fever diagnosis?

2 major

Or

1 major & two minor

What are the *minor* (Jones) criteria?	Fever
	Arthralgia
	Prolonged P-R interval
	Prior rheumatic fever or heart disease
	Elevated acute-phase reactants (ESR/CRP, leukocytes, etc.)
If you suspect rheumatic fever, and obtain a throat culture, what is the likely outcome?	Cultures are usually negative by the time rheumatic fever has developed
If your patient presents with strep throat, & you do a rapid Strep test (rapid antigen detection test), what should you know about the sensitivity & specificity of the test?	The specificity is good! (>95 %)
	The sensitivity is just moderate, though (around 75 %) – so get a throat culture also, even if negative!
Why is it important to isolate the Strep organism involved in a Strep throat infection? (2 reasons)	To confirm the Strep infection
	To type the organism (more information about the risk for rheumatic fever, etc.)
Which serological tests are useful to support a diagnosis of rheumatic fever, & when should you be able to obtain a positive result?	There are many – most common are ASO (antistreptolysin O), anti-DNase B, antihyaluronidase, antistreptokinase
	They rise in the first month after Strep infection & should be present if rheumatic fever is present
When does ASO titer peak, & how sensitive is it?	2–3 weeks after rheumatic fever onset Sensitivity about 85 %
Is group A Strep the only one that produces elevated ASO titers?	No – Groups C & G do, too
What does GBS cause in pregnant mothers?	UTIs + asymptomatic colonization of the vagina/anus
Is group B Strep a likely cause of meningitis occurring in the first 7 days of life?	**No – it usually causes septicemia & pneumonia in the "early-onset" period**

Early-onset GBS is especially likely to affect which infants?	– Premature – Mom had obstetrical complications
"Late-late"-onset GBS infection occurs at what age?	>3 months
Which infants typically develop late-late-onset GBS?	Preemies who have, or used to have, IV lines
What kind of infection does late-late-onset GBS usually cause, and how bad is it?	– Bacteremia without a focus – <1 % fatality rate
When is GBS most likely to cause meningitis?	Late onset (7 days – 3 months)
What percentage of meningitis in children 7 days to 3 months old is due to GBS?	40 %
Which GBS serotype is usually involved in late-onset GBS infection?	TYPE III (90 %) Mnemonic: 3 months – Type III
If an infant develops meningitis in the first week of life, is it very likely to be GBS meningitis?	No
Osteomyelitis is typically caused by Staph aureus. For what age group is this *not true*, and what is the common organism?	– 7 days to 3 months (late-onset GBS) – GBS
What is the gold standard for diagnosing GBS infection in infants?	Positive blood culture
Can antigens be used to diagnose GBS infection?	Yes – <u>only if</u> 1. infant has been on antibiotics 2. serum or CSF is used
Which body fluid *must not* be used to diagnose GBS infection? (based on antigens)	<u>Urine</u> (not at all reliable)

If GBS causes osteomyelitis or septic arthritis, how should you treat that?	4-week IV antibiotics (usually PCN)
IV treatment of serious GBS infections usually begins with what drug combo?	IV PCN + gentamicin
How long is the treatment regimen for pneumonia/sepsis due to GBS?	10 days (Start with PCN + gent, then just PCN)
How long is the treatment regimen for GBS meningitis?	14 days minimum
So, if an infant is diagnosed with GBS osteomyelitis, what is the treatment regimen?	IV PCN + gentamicin initially, then IV PCN ×4 weeks
How is the treatment regimen different for GBS sepsis and GBS meningitis, compared to GBS septic arthritis or osteomyelitis?	Same drugs, but meningitis is 14 days (minimum), sepsis is 10 days, arthritis is 4 weeks
Which enterococci infect humans?	*E. faecalis and E. faecium*
Enteroccocal infections are most often seen in which pediatric patient group?	Newborns (UTI, abdominal infection, bacteremia)
Enterococci are particularly fond of infecting which sorts of foreign objects in the body?	VP shunts in kids (meningitis & ventriculitis) Indwelling urinary catheters Central venous lines in neonates
Enterococcal neonatal sepsis has increased over the last 30 years. How common is it as a cause of neonatal bactermia & sepsis?	Roughly 10 % (according to most recent data available)
Which enterococcus causes most neonatal infection?	*E. faecalis*
How are enterococci treated?	PCN or ampicillin if sensitive
Why is it so important to check sensitivities on enterococcal infections?	To identify vanc-resistant enterococcus (VRE)

If a boards question asks whether you would like to get sensitivities on an enterococcal infection, what is the correct answer?

Yes
(they want to know you are aware of VRE)

If a boards question offers you a 3rd-generation cephalosporin to treat enterococcus, is that a reasonable choice?
(*Popular test item!*)

<u>No</u> – it will not treat enterococcus

What can you use to treat VRE?

Linezolid or daptomycin

If an enterococcal infection is sensitive to ampicillin, why might you choose to add a medication to the ampicillin regimen?

For <u>synergy</u> in bad infections, an aminoglycoside will help to kill enterococci, rather than just inhibit their growth

(Amp & PCN are *static* antibiotics against most enterococci!)

If your patient has an enterococcal UTI, what should you check?

US for underlying abnormalities – enterococcal UTIs are associated with a higher than usual rate of underlying urinary tract abnormalities

Which peds patients are at risk for Listeria infections?

Mainly newborns
(+ any institutionalized patient)

Where do infected newborns encounter Listeria?

Colonized moms

In the environment, where might your patients contact Listeria?

Sheep, goats, poultry, & *contaminated milk products*

What is an especially classic exposure for Listeria?
(*popular test item*)

Goat cheese from California or Mexico!

If Listeria appears in a blood or a CSF culture, should you consider it a possible contaminant?

No
(not in a kid <3 months old, at least)

Can you treat Listeria with a 3rd-generation cephalosporin?

No
(Listeria & enterococcus are treated with ampicillin!)

If your patient is "penicillin allergic," how can you treat a Listeria infection?	Vanc or TMP/SMX
If a blood or a CSF culture comes back as "diphtheroid" organism, should you figure it's a contaminant? If not, why not?	– No – That is the initial designation for Listeria (before the specific identification is made)
Which bacterium causes the disease diphtheria?	Corynebacterium
What are the hallmarks of diphtheria?	– **Hoarse with sore throat** – **Low-grade temp** – **Gray-white pharyngeal membrane**
What is the most worrisome complication in diphtheria infection, other than the respiratory compromise issues? (*popular test item!*)	**Myocarditis**
How is diphtheria treated?	Antibiotics (PCN or erythro) + *Antitoxin*
On the boards, a patient who presents with diphtheria will typically be in what demographic group?	An immigrant (sometimes from Eastern Europe) (*idea being that immigrants may not have been immunized*)
What are the two main complications of diphtheria, other than airway issues?	1. myocarditis 2. polyneuritis
What are the two infectious diseases for which treatment with antitoxin is crucial?	Diphtheria + tetanus (*patient will not get better without it!*)
What kind of infection does arcanobacterium cause?	Pharyngitis (like GAS) + scarlet fever rash

Are there any important complications related to arcanobacterium infections?	<u>No</u>
What treats arcanobacterium infections?	Almost anything! – PCN, erythro, tetracycline, etc.
A black eschar on the skin of a farm kid = what diagnosis?	(cutaneous) anthrax
Are the skin lesions of anthrax infection painful?	No (draining lymph nodes may be)
What three forms can anthrax infection take?	Cutaneous (95 %) Pulmonic (near 5 % – aka inhalational) GI
Is anthrax infection only seen in bioterrorism incidents?	No! It occurs in nature, especially with livestock contact (usually cutaneous), consumption of infected animals (GI), and inhalation due to work with contaminated wool. Skins, or bone meal (inhalational)
Do you need to notify anyone if you see a case of suspected anthrax (in the US)?	Yes, it is a reportable disease – Notify local health authorities & the CDC (If bioterrorism *is* a concern, notify FBI via local police)
What is the big difference in treatment regimens between naturally acquired anthrax, and anthrax contracted through bioterrorism?	Penicillin/amoxicillin is the drug of choice(!) for naturally occurring anthrax Treatment must still be rapid, but fancy medication regimens are not needed
If you are treating an anthrax patient with systemic involvement with penicillin, what type of dosing must you use?	Meningitis level – Meningitis is often a component of systemic anthrax, so PCN penetration of the blood–brain barrier is important!

Is it safe to begin anthrax treatment with penicillin or amoxicillin, if bioterror is not suspected?

No –
Current pediatric guidelines recommend beginning with ciprofloxacin (change to PCN or amoxicillin if susceptible when test results are available)

Is anthrax pneumonia communicable from ordinary person-to-person contact?

No
(plague pneumonia is though, <u>big time</u>)

A young military recruit presents with what seems like pneumonia. On CXR, you see a widened mediastinum. Diagnosis?

Pneumonia + wide mediastinum = *anthrax pneumonia*

If a patient has just been exposed to anthrax, how can you decontaminate him or her, so that others aren't infected?

Spores remaining on the patient or patient's clothes can infect others. Remove clothing & decontaminate patient with soap & water

For children & adults, what is the drug of choice for uncomplicated cases of cutaneous or GI anthrax, *if the source of anthrax exposure might be aerosol (such as in a bioterror attack)*?

Ciprofloxacin or doxycycline

(60 days, as usual)

Why is the treatment length so long, when inhalational anthrax is possible?

Because spores stuck in the lung sometimes don't start growing for a long time after they are inhaled –

The 60 days is to try to be sure antibiotic is present if they do!

Why is anthrax vaccination recommended for patients with pulmonary anthrax or inhaled exposure to anthrax?

The same reason –
Just in case a spore sits in the lung a long time before starting to develop, the body's immune system would be ready

What is the issue, currently, with immunizing children following an aerosol anthrax exposure?

The vaccine is not yet (as of 2014) FDA approved for children – informed consent required to administer it

How do you treat uncomplicated cutaneous anthrax in kids if you have no suspicions of bioterror?

Ciprofloxacin or doxycycline –

7–10-day treatment course

(may use PCN or amoxicillin if susceptibility is good – but resistance can develop during monotherapy treatment)

For a very systemic anthrax infection, such as pulmonary anthrax, what medication should you use initially?

Ciprofloxacin & clindamycin

(Idea is to combine a cidal antibiotic with a protein inhibitor antibiotic – if sensitive, can change to PCN, doxycycline, etc., later)

What medications are recommended, in addition to the core fluoroquinolone medication, for treatment of systemic anthrax infections?

Clindamycin & doxycycline

Rifampin &
Linezolid

What is the difference between the duration of treatment for the systemic infection, and the duration of post-exposure prophylaxis?

Prophylaxis is *always 60 days*!

Treatment is shorter, until resolution of infection
(10 days for cutaneous,
usually 14 days for systemic)

Anthrax can sometimes cause meningitis. If anthrax meningitis is suspected, what commonly used anthrax antibiotic should you AVOID?

Doxycycline –
It doesn't cross the blood–brain barrier well

What treatment is recommended for systemic anthrax WITH meningitis?

Ciprofloxacin +
Meropenem +
Linezolid

Minimum 2–3-weeks duration!

(Idea is to combine
one quinolone with
one beta lactam or glycopeptide &
one protein synthesis inhibitor)

Which antibiotic is preferred for a pregnant or breast feeding mother, who may have been exposed to anthrax?

Amoxicillin or Clindamycin –
Consider others depending on susceptibilities & risk vs. benefit

Children living on a military base present with painless skin lesions, and two have a cough/tachypnea. What is it?

Anthrax exposure due to bioterrorism

If inhalational anthrax *exposure* is suspected in a pediatric patient, what treatment regimen should be given, and for how long?

Ciprofloxacin –
60 days

(even for preemies . . .)

What special treatment can be obtained from the CDC, if inhalational anthrax is suspected, in addition to the usual antibiotics?

Raxibacumab – a monoclonal antibody

(can also be used as prophylaxis, if other therapies cannot be)

Is cutaneous anthrax communicable due to person-to-person contact?

No

(*rare cases of transmission from body fluid contact at lesion sites may occur*)

What CXR finding do you look for to identify pulmonary anthrax?

Wide mediastinum

What is the unusual shape of the anthrax organism, if micro information is provided?

They look like "boxcars" from a train, all lined up!

A patient presents with nausea & vomiting after eating Chinese food that was left out for a while. What is the organism and treatment?

– *Bacillus cereus*
– No treatment

If you're eating rice infested with *B. cereus*, how do you know whether you'll get vomiting vs. diarrhea?

– if the bacteria hasn't had time to make toxin yet, you get diarrhea because it makes the toxin in your gut (8–16-h incubation time)
– if toxin was already made and in the food, you start vomiting within a few hours

Will cooking the food better protect you from the emetic form of *B. cereus* toxicity?

No – the toxin is heat stable

Normally, we think of *B. cereus* with fried rice "food poisoning." What two unusual infections is it also able to produce?

1. IV catheter infection
2. Eye infection after penetrating globe injury

How are serious *B. cereus* infections treated?   **Vancomycin**

Profuse diarrhea in a hospitalized patient who has recently been treated with an antibiotic = what diagnosis?   *C. difficile*

Can vancomycin be given orally?   Yes

How does *Clostridium perfringens* cause problems for the gut?   24-h diarrhea – rapid onset

If you suspect that a patient has *C. difficile* colitis, how do you diagnose it by labs?   *C. diff* toxin (not culture) –

FYI: False negatives are common

What is the first line treatment for *C. difficile* colitis?   Metronidazole <u>*PO*</u>

If a boards question discusses a patient with palpable purpura, and a state (such as North Carolina) is mentioned, what is the diagnosis?   RMSF
(Rocky Mountain spotted fever)

If a patient is presented who is ill, has petechiae + hypotension, and <u>no state</u> is mentioned, what is the diagnosis?   *Neisseria meningitidis*/bacteremia

Which patients *do not* need any treatment after possible tetanus exposure?   <5 years since last tetanus

If a patient sustains a "clean" wound, and had a tetanus immunization 6–10 years ago, is any treatment required?   No – within 10 years is alright for clean wounds

When should tetanus IG be given?
(2 situations)   Dirty wound +
1. <3 tetanus immunizations completed
2. immunization history unknown

If a pregnant woman is exposed to N. meningitis, should she have Rifampin prophylaxis?   <u>No</u> –
Rifampin is contraindicated in pregnancy
(use ceftriaxone)

If Gram-negative diplococci are seen in the vaginal discharge of a female patient, can it be normal flora?	Yes – Females sometimes have other Neisseria species as normal flora – doesn't have to be *N. gonorrhoeae*
How should you conclusively diagnose *N. gonorrhoeae* in a female patient?	Culture (but treat anyway if suspicion is high)
Are Gram-negative diplococci ever seen as normal flora in male patients?	No – it's gonorrhea
Special susceptibility to *N. meningitidis* infection is associated with what immune system problem?	Complement deficiency (and asplenia)
Moraxella catarrhalis frequently causes what two infections?	1. Otitis media 2. Sinusitis
What is special about *M. catarrhalis*?	B-lactamase producer (susceptible to most other antibiotics)
Pseudomonas is famous for causing what infection in diabetics?	Chronic otitis externa
A neutropenic patient presents with little round raised lesions, dark, with a central ulcer. What is the lesion called, and what caused it?	– Ecthyma gangrenosum – Pseudomonas
If a patient sustains a puncture wound to the foot, through a rubber-soled shoe, what is the organism to watch for?	Pseudomonas
If a diffuse red rash develops around hair follicles, and the patient has a history of hot tub use, what is it and how do you treat it?	– Hot tub folliculitis (pseudomonas) – No treatment needed
If a patient presents who is infected with a "Burkholderia" species, what underlying disorder should you suspect the patient has?	CF (cystic fibrosis)

There are two types of Burkholderia. How were they previously designated? (In other words, why haven't you ever heard of them before?)

They *were* pseudomonas species – recent change

In general, what is the significance of a Burkholderia infection?

Bad prognostic + difficult to treat

Patients with turtles or other reptiles at home, who develop diarrhea, have what diagnosis?

Salmonella (usually non-typhi)

Iguana + diarrhea =

Salmonella infection

In addition to reptiles, where else does Salmonella exposure occur?

Eggs/chickens and milk

Homemade Thanksgiving stuffing & a family diarrhea outbreak = what organism?

Salmonella (grandma put raw eggs in the stuffing!)

Typhoid fever has what two recognizable signs that *S. typhi* is the cause of the diarrhea?

– "Rose spots" on trunk 1 week after fever starts (light red macules)
– Low WBCs

Who was "Typhoid Mary" and why is she important to your peds boards?

– **A food handler who spread a lot of typhoid**
– **She reminds us that Salmonella species sometimes cause an asymptomatic carrier state**

If your patient will be traveling to someplace with a lot of typhoid, what should you recommend?

Oral typhoid vaccine (must be older than 2 years to take it)

If a child presents with high fever, seizure and diarrhea, and has a bandemia on labs, what is the diagnosis?

Shigella

A child in or from the developing world presents with rectal prolapse during a febrile diarrheal illness. What is the infection?

Shigella

(diarrhea + rectal prolapse in the US is usually trichuria aka "whipworm")

Most childhood diarrheal illnesses can be treated with TMP/SMX, if antibiotic treatment is indicated. Will this work for Shigella?

No – it is usually resistant – Use a 3rd-generation cephalosporin or azithromycin

Is Pepto-Bismol® a good way to treat or prevent traveller's diarrhea in kids?
(bismuth subsalicylate)

**No –
it contains lots of salicylate**
(aspirin-type toxicity!)

When dealing with *E. coli* diarrhea, why is it important to know whether the causative organism is ETEC (traveller's diarrhea) or EHEC (hemorrhagic diarrhea)?

Antibiotic treatment improves ETEC, but *increases* probability of HUS in EHEC!

What clue from the microbiology lab tells you that you are dealing with EHEC? (a clue you would never normally know!)

It only grows with "<u>sorbitol-enhanced agar</u>"

Mnemonic: Imagine bloody sugar cubes sitting on an agar plate

What is the triad of HUS, and which diarrheal illness is it associated with?

1. **Renal failure**
2. **Hemolytic anemia**
3. **Thrombocytopenia**
   E. coli **0157:H7**

What is the other acronym for EHEC?

STEC (Shiga-toxin-producing *E. coli*)

Epidemic *E. coli* outbreaks are famous for occurring in what two settings?

1. Undercooked beef
2. Waterpark outbreak

Less well-known sources for EHEC infection are what two foods?

1. Unpasteurized milk
2. Apple juice

If a vignette mentions that a child has not had their immunizations, or the parents refused childhood immunizations, what infection should you (mainly) worry about?

H. flu

You have done a bacteremia work-up, and the blood culture comes back positive for *H. flu*. You call the family & the child is doing fine – what should you do?

<u>Treat</u> it!

***H. flu* bacteremia is <u>always</u> treated**

(Strep pneumo bacteremia is *not* treated if the kid is fine)

What is the buzzword for *H. flu* on micro?

"Pleomorphic" Gram-negative coccobacillus

With *H. flu* meningitis, should you give steroids automatically?

Yes – it reduces hearing loss & other neuro sequelae

How do you treat *H. flu* bacteremia?

Admit for IV ceftriaxone

A child with a red & prominently swollen cheek presents to you. You can feel the margins of the rash when you palpate the inner surface of the cheek. What is this?

Buccal cellulitis
(often *H. flu*,
often a picture on the boards,
vanishingly rare now with *H. flu*
immunization)

H. flu has historically been known for causing what throat disorder?

Epiglottitis –
with a "cherry red" epiglottis

Do contacts of a patient with a significant (meaning not OM) *H. flu* infection require chemoprophylaxis?

Yes, if <4 years old & not fully immunized OR immunocompromised

(Rifampin × 4 days for household contacts)

Why might a patient with *H. flu* also require "chemoprophylaxis"?

Therapeutic antibiotics do not always eradicate carriage of *H. flu*, so if susceptible household members are present they would still be at risk from the patient

How is plague transmitted?

Bite of infected fleas

A young person presents with a hemorrhagic pneumonia "spewing blood" on the boards exam. What is the likely boards diagnosis?

Pulmonic plague (bioterrorism in most cases)

Is pulmonic plague contagious from person-to-person regular contact?

Highly!
(due to coughing)

Is it a good idea to aspirate the swollen lymph node, if plague is suspected? What about in a cat scratch disease?

Plague – yes (for diagnosis)

Cat Scratch – no
(can lead to fistulas)

Mnemonic: it is never a good idea to stick a needle in a cat!

Is bubonic plague a big problem, in terms of mortality/morbidity?

No –
It's the pneumonic form that's so deadly

A patient presents with RLQ pain & rebound, and appears to have appendicitis. The lab notifies you that an organism has been identified from one of the bodily fluids. What is the organism?

(Popular test item!)

Yersinia enterocolitica

There are two related organisms that cause a "pseudoappendicitis" presentation. What are they?

(Popular test item!)

Yersinia enterocolitica

&

Yersinia pseudotuberculosis

Patients with too much iron (due to transfusions, hemochromatosis, etc.) are likely to become bacteremic with what organism?

(Popular test item!)

Yersinia enterocolitica

(it has a special interest in iron)

Chitlins (the food) + diarrhea =

Yersinia enterocolitica **infection**

Iron overload patient + bacteremia =

Probable *Y. enterocolitica* **infection**

Sickle cell patients are generally anemic, but can a sickle cell patient also be iron overloaded?

Yes –
Due to hemolysis + transfusions

Legionella can be treated with erythromycin, but it requires a high-dose regimen. If a child treated with e-mycin develops hearing loss, is it the e-mycin or the Legionella that did it?

(Popular test item!)

The erythromycin
(at high doses)

(IV azithromycin is the drug of choice, though, for pediatric Legionella)

Atypical pneumonia + diarrhea, often accompanied by hyponatremia, is what disorder?

Legionella pneumonia

Klebsiella mainly causes pneumonia + UTIs. What is important to know about it?

Always β-lactam resistant (Moraxella, also)

What medication(s) treat(s) tularemia?

Streptomycin

Or

Doxycycline

If a boards question has streptomycin as an answer option, you should go back to see whether the question is actually dealing with which two disorders?

Resistant TB

Or

Tularemia

How do patients usually contract tularemia?

Tick bites

(other types of animal contact can also produce infection, at times, including rabbit skinning)

How do you diagnose tularemia?

By serology –
do <u>not</u> aspirate nodes

What weird complication of cat scratch disease sometimes occurs, but spontaneously resolves?

Encephalitis/seizures

If you're not supposed to aspirate cat scratch nodes (don't stick needles into cats, remember), how do you make the diagnosis?

Either clinically or serology

Should cat scratch fever be treated?

Optional –
azithromycin may "speed resolution"

Citrobacter is associated with what type of infection?

Brain abscess

(*Popular test item!*)

If a neonate with a fever has Citrobacter in the blood culture, what test(s) should you order next?

LP (if not already done)

+

Head CT

Low sodium + history of tick bite =	RMSF
A child who is less than 8 years old develops RMSF. How should you treat him/her on the boards?	Chloramphenicol (often can't get in real world – use doxycyline)
The evolution of the RMSF rash is? (2 aspects)	1. Maculopapular to petechial 2. Centripetal – begins distally & works inward Mnemonic: Remember, you injure your palms & soles climbing rocky mountains
What is the usual treatment for RMSF?	Doxycycline
How do patients contract RMSF?	Tick bite
Where can patients contract RMSF?	*Not* in the Rocky Mountains – New England to Texas (skipping Florida & Louisiana)
What is Rocky Mountain spot<u>less</u> fever? (*Popular test item!*)	**Ehrlichiosis** (same fever & arthralgias-usually no rash)
There are two forms of Ehrlichiosis- what's the difference? (*Popular test item!*)	**One lives in monocytes, the other lives in neutrophils**
Which form of Ehrlichiosis affects granulocytes, and is typically a dog Ehrlichiosis pathogen – now identified also in humans?	*Ehrlichia ewingii*
A flu-like illness with pancytopenia and a "morula" on the smear = (*Popular test item!*)	**Ehrlichiosis** (tick-borne) (*morula refers to a "berry-like" cluster of intracellular organisms*)
Where is Ehrlichiosis found? **(geographically)** (*Popular test item!*)	**Same distribution as Lyme disease + West coast & near Great Lakes**

An adenitis that does not respond to the usual antibiotics is probably due to what sort of organism?   Mycobacteria

(*Popular test item!*)

How is mycobacterial adenitis treated?   **Excise entire node**

(*Popular test item!*)

A child develops skin ulcerations in a line on his arm after straining to reach into an aquarium to feed his fish. What is this?   *M. marinum*
(tracks along lymphatics)

(*Popular test item!*)

Lymphatic infection + fish tank or fresh water pool =   *M. marinum* **infection**

(*Popular test item!*)

How are children usually exposed to tuberculosis?   By adults

How does tuberculosis usually manifest itself in children?   Usually it doesn't! (asymptomatic)

Does TB usually cause pulmonary infection during the primary infection?   **No –**
But if it does, the problem is usually in the <u>lower</u> lobe (not upper lobe)

What usually happens after the primary TB infection resolves?   It goes into a latent phase – May reactivate later in the upper lobe

Obvious pulmonary infection with primary TB occurs most often in which patients?   Adolescents
&
HIV infected

When dealing with fluid related to tuberculosis (pleural or pericardial effusion), how useful is a sample of the fluid for making the TB diagnosis?   Not very –
Biopsy of nearby tissue is better

On neuroimaging, what findings suggest TB meningitis?   Enhancement of basal ganglia/posterior areas
(+ *pus at the base of the brain*)

Clinically, what findings suggest TB meningitis, as opposed to other types of meningitis?

Slow, chronic course

+

Cranial nerve findings
(due to pus accumulating at base of brain)

What electrolyte/endocrine problem often occurs with TB meningitis?

SIADH
(hyponatremia)

Is meningitis a common development for people infected with TB?

No –
Only common on the boards

When adolescents present with TB, it is often reactivation disease. How do they present?

(three categories of symptoms – generalized pulmonary radiological)

1. Generalized symptoms: fever, wt loss, night sweats
2. Pulmonary: cough, hemoptysis, pleuritic chest pain
3. Radiological: upper lobe infiltrate with hilar LAD

In other words, they have the classic TB presentation!

What is the problem with placing a PPD on a 4-month-old infant?

(Popular test item!)

Not reliable for infants <6 months old

After exposure to TB, how long does it take for the PPD to turn positive, if the patient has contracted the disease?

(Popular test item!)

About 3 months

When is it alright to place a PPD, in relation to a possible TB exposure?

(Popular test item!)

**Anytime –
but you will need to repeat it after 3 months have elapsed to be sure**

(You still want to test early, because if it is positive, you will start treatment)

What determines whether the PPD is positive or not?

Amount of induration

(Color of the skin is <u>irrelevant!</u>)

How large does the PPD site need to be for you to consider it positive? (generally speaking)

15 mm

Patients in what age group have a lesser requirement for judging their PPD to be positive?

Kids <4 years old are considered positive at 10 mms

Usually, 15 mm of induration is needed to consider a PPD test positive. For which patient groups is 10 mm sufficient?

Kids <4 years old

&

Anyone you'd be concerned about (*health care workers, institutionalized people, homeless, diabetic, immigrants,* etc.)

If a patient is PPD positive, what should you do about it?

Get a CXR and sputum to check for active disease

If your patient is PPD positive, but you don't find any active disease, how should you treat him or her?

6–9 months of INH

If you evaluate a PPD-positive patient, and find active disease, how should you treat him or her?

4 drug therapy until sensitivities come back (*multidrug-resistant TB is a very ugly problem*)

What four drugs are in the "four-drug TB regimen?"

INH
Rifampin
Pyrazinamide
Ethambutol or streptomycin

Mnemonic:
The drugs can be rearranged to spell SPIRE-like the sharp tip of a tower skewering a TB "red snapper"

Why are TB bugs called "red snappers?"

They are acid-fast on stain, so they look bright red

For which patients could 5 mms of induration on the PPD be considered positive?
                    (2 groups)

– seriously immuno-compromised

(*HIV or other T-cell disorders, organ transplant patient, chronic high-dose steroids*)

– or seriously worried

(*bad lung disease/fibrosis, close contact with case*)

What is the name of the stuff used for the PPD?

(Popular test item!)

Mantoux 5 Todd units

There is a certain patient group for whom you should *not* prescribe ethambutol. What group is it?

Children too young to be tested for color vision

Why is color vision testing important for patients taking ethambutol?

Its main side effect is decreasing visual acuity, and loss of color vision is the first sign that this side effect is developing

What is the main side effect of the three core anti-TB drugs?
(INH, rifampin, & pyrazinamide)

Hepatotoxicity
(all three of them do it)

Should routine testing for hepatotoxicity be conducted when giving INH, rifampin, and/or pyrazinamide?
(Popular test item!)

No –
Testing is <u>only indicated</u> if symptoms of liver trouble develop

Sulfur-colored granules coming from a facial abscess = what diagnosis?
Known question of interest

Actinomyces infection

What unusual pathogen is sometimes involved in PID if an IUD is in place?

Actinomyces (yuck!)

What kills actinomyces?

Gram+ antibiotics
(including PCN)

What have Chlamydia species been redesignated?

Chlamydophila (!)

Where do *Chlamydia psittaci* infections come from?

Birds – especially in the house

What is the hallmark of *Chlamydia psittaci* pneumonia?
Known question of interest

Pneumonia <u>with splenomegaly</u>

Are *Chlamydia psittaci* pneumonia patients ill appearing?

Yes, definitely

(Rigors, high temp, myalgias – not like "walking pneumonia")

Does Chlamydia pneumoniae infection come from birds?

No –
It's spread person-to-person

Are *Chlamydia pneumoniae* patients usually very ill?

No –
wheezing is common, but not very ill

What kind of Chlamydia sometimes causes pneumonia in young infants?

Trachomatis

Which type of Chlamydia causes eye infection in newborns?

Trachomatis

What is the classic presentation of chlamydia pneumonia in infants?

Afebrile infant with a "staccato cough"

A child presents with fever, headache, increased LFTs. The history involves exposure to pet mammals and water that the animals have been in or near. What is the diagnosis?

Leptospirosis

What is the connection between the animals, water, and leptospirosis infection?

Leptospirosis from the animal's urine gets into the water

How do you make the diagnosis of leptospirosis (conclusively)?

Blood culture

(serological tests to assist with rapid diagnosis are sometimes available, but begin treatment on clinical suspicion if they are not!)

If the organism is in the urine, why can't I just culture the urine?

(Known question of interest)

It is in the urine, but not until very late in the course

If a leukemia patient develops line sepsis, and cultures show Candida, what should you do?

Known question of interest

Pull the line
&
Start amphotericin B

For any significantly sick patient with a fungal infection, what should you do?

Known question of interest

Start Ampho B (IV)

What skin disorder does Malassezia furfur cause?

Tinea versicolor
(lesions fluoresce with Woods lamp)

What does M. furfur look like on a KOH prep?

Spaghetti 'n' meatballs!

Why is it hard to get rid of Tinea versicolor?

It is normal human flora

What are the important predisposing factors for development of Tinea versicolor?

Sweating & high cortisol levels

(That's why it so often develops in *adolescents* – they tend to be sweaty with high cortisol levels)

What systemic treatment is helpful if your patient is really motivated to treat a widespread tinea infection?

Ketoconazole –
It's excreted in the sweat

(the other "azole" medications are also effective)

If a vignette indicates that the patient is a *very* low birth weight infant on lipid hyperalimentation, and the patient is infected with something, what is it?

Malassezia furfur
(it has a thing for lipids – just like *Yersinia enterocolitica* has a thing for iron!)

(*Known question of interest*)

What is the giveaway that your patient has a Malassezia furfur infection, in terms of the micro info?
Known question of interest

Olive oil overlay is needed to grow out the blood culture
(in addition to Sabouraud's medium)

If your patient has an invasive *M. furfur* infection, what is the correct treatment?
(3 things to think about)

- **Pull the lines**
- **D/C lipid infusion**
- **Ampho B (1 mg/kg/day)**

Pneumonia + splenomegaly = what diagnosis?

Chlamydia psittaci pneumonia

If an adolescent patient isn't responding to over-the-counter treatment for athlete's foot (Tinea pedis), then what is the likely problem?

Candida
(the "azole" topicals, like miconazole, will kill both)

Which patient group is most likely to develop Tinea pedis (athlete's foot)?

Adolescent males

An adolescent patient with AIDS presents with meningitis on your board exam. What unusual pathogen is likely?	*Cryptococcus*
How is *cryptococcus* diagnosed? (two methods)	Cyroptococcal antigen <u>or</u> "India ink" preparation (has a big halo around it)
Does cryptococcal meningitis usually present with a chronic or rapid onset?	Chronic
A child has been helping his grandmother in the garden. He develops an ulcerated lesion on one fingertip. What is the problem? *(Known question of interest)*	**Sporothrix**
What are the treatment options for Sporothrix?	**Itraconazole** **Or** **A saturated solution of potassium iodide** **(both are taken <u>PO</u>!)**
A diabetic adolescent presents with black eschar in, or on, the nose. What is it, and how is it treated? Known question of interest	• **Invasive mucormycosis. It is <u>bad</u>.** • **Treat with extensive debridement + Ampho B**
Where does invasive mucormycosis begin?	**Nasal turbinates or hard palate** *(remember: black eschar)*
Which patients are at risk for invasive mucormycosis?	Immunocompromised (*including diabetics – the fugus is everywhere in soil, bread, etc.*)
Is eosinophilia a hallmark of protozoal disease?	<u>No</u> – that's parasites
If a patient is infected, and the question involves a kitty litter box, what is the infection? *(Popular test item!)*	**Toxoplasmosis**
Diarrhea following berry eating = infection by what organism? *(Popular test item!)*	**Cyclospora**

How is cyclospora infection treated?

TMP/SMX
(Bactrim®)

Which two diarrhea causing organisms are "acid-fast?"

Cyclospora

&

Cryptosporidium

What is unusual about cryptosporididum infections?

(*Popular test item!*)

Tends to be epidemic

&

**Watery diarrhea lasts
1–2 weeks!**

In the immunocompromised, what is different about cryptosporidial infection?

(*Popular test item!*)

The infection becomes chronic & requires treatment (nitazoxanide is the first line)

In infectious disease, "maltese crosses" go with what disorder?

Babesiosis

(they clump together & form the shape of a Maltese Cross)

Which patients with a specific sort of immunocompromise are in especially bad trouble if they contract malaria?

Asplenic patients!

If you have a malaria blood smear with multiple RBCs infected in one field or multiple parasites are in each RBC, what type of malaria are you dealing with?

(*Popular test item!*)

P. falciparum (**the really dangerous one**)

Mnemonic: Think of it as "Fancy-parum" – it's the one that creates the really "fancy" complications

Which type of malaria has only been identified in the last few years, and produces severe infections very similar to falciparum?

P. knowlesi

(found in Southeast Asia)

On the peds boards, if they show a malaria blood smear & you're not sure what it shows, what should you guess?

(*Popular test item!*)

P. falciparum (it's the main one they want you to know about)

Is chloroquine usually good malaria treatment/prophylaxis?

(*Popular test item!*)

No –
Most malaria is resistant

(must check for each geographical region)

If your patient is traveling to Africa or Asia, what should you assume when deciding on their malaria prophylaxis regimen?

Assume the malaria is chloroquine resistant

If your patient is traveling to an area where the malaria is <u>definitely</u> chloroquine sensitive, what prophylaxis regimen should you prescribe?

Chloroquine!

(We don't want to encourage resistance in the few areas where it's still effective.)

If a malaria patient is too ill to take meds PO, what should you do?

Give IV artesunate
(an artemisinin drug available from the CDC)

(IV quinidine is also an option, but studies indicate the newer artesunate reduces both mortality & complications)

Should the dangerous falciparum or knowlesi malaria be treated with IV monotherapy?

A second agent (generally oral) should be added to improve efficacy & reduce relapses

Cerebral malaria is when the malaria affects the brain, causing seizures. Are steroids helpful for cerebral malaria?

<u>No</u>
(don't give – could make things worse)

What is the most important thing to remember about malaria prophylaxis?

Take it
<u>before,</u>
<u>during,</u>
<u>and after</u> the trip

Which two types of malaria sometimes take up prolonged residence in the liver?

Vivax + ovale
Mnemonic:
Vodka goes to the liver – v & o are the first 2 letters of vodka, reminding you that these two stay in the liver.

Should chloroquine ever be used to treat *P. falciparum*?

(*Popular test item!*)

No

Which medication gets rid of the hypnozoites, the malaria forms that live long-term in the liver?

Primaquine

Why don't the other meds kill the forms living in the liver?

The other meds only kill <u>free</u> organisms – if it's hidden inside a cell (including RBCs) they can't get to it

If a question asks about a particular site that some malaria use to attach to the RBC, what is the name of the site?

The "Duffy antigen" site

(Vivax malaria)

(*Popular test item!*)

Which of the four types of malaria is most associated with <u>nephritic syndrome</u>?

P. malariae

(all types are associated with nephritis, in general)

(*Popular test item!*)

Where should you look for a "Maltese Cross" in a Babesia infection?

Inside the RBC

A patient who has visited the Northeastern USA presents with cyclic fevers, hemoglobinuria, anemia, and emotional lability. What's the problem?

Babesiosis

Where does Babesiosis come from?

Ticks –
Often co-infected with Lyme or Ehrlichiosis

If a patient presents with anemia, pancytopenia, cyclic fever, & rigors, on the boards, what's wrong with him or her?

Babesiosis <u>with</u> Ehrlichiosis coinfection (hence the pancytopenia)

(*Popular test item!*)

How is babesiosis treated?

Clindamycin + quinine (usually)

In mild cases of babesiosis, or in treatment failures, what other antibiotic treatment regimen is recommended?

Atovaquone & azithromycin

(has fewer side effects than the Clinda + quinine regimen, also)

A child living in Texas, near the border of Mexico, presents with a liver abscess. What is it likely to be, and how do you diagnose it? (*Popular test item!*)	– *Entamoeba histolytica* – Serology – *don't* aspirate it!
How is *Entamoeba histolytica* infection treated?	Metronidazole (or tinidazole) + Paromomycin or diloxanide (used to clear the organisms in the gut, which are *not* killed by the systemic treatment)
In the USA, which patients are at risk of developing amebiasis? **(4 groups)**	– **US residents living near the border of Mexico** – **Immigrants** – **Gay men** – **Institutionalized patients**
Who gets Giardia in the USA (usually)? **(4 groups)**	1. **Campers** 2. **Returning travelers** 3. **Daycare kids** 4. **Immunoglobulin (Ig) disorders**
What are the giveaways for Giardia infection, in terms of symptoms? (*Known question of interest*)	**Flatulence & distension** & **watery, smelly, uncontrollable diarrhea**
In some cases, Giardia can become a chronic infection. If this happens, what are the main symptoms? **(3)** (*Popular test item!*)	1. **Flatulence** 2. **Soft stools** 3. **"Sulfuric" belching (eructation)**
Where does Giardia live (in the human body)?	In the duodenum
How is it transmitted?	Fecal-oral (*especially from beavers & muskrats!*)

How is *Entamoeba histolytica* transmitted?

Fecal-oral

How is Giardia treated, or will it spontaneously resolve?

It's usually severe enough (& contagious enough) that it should be treated –

Use metronidazole or tinidazole

How is the diagnosis of Giardia made, based on labs?

(3 ways)

1. Giardia specific antigen (in stool)
2. Fresh stool O & P
3. String test

Although the string test only occurs on the boards, you should know how it is done. What is the procedure?

A string is swallowed – long enough to end up in the duodenum – while the remainder stays exterior. Giardia adhere to the string, which is microscopically inspected after is it taken out.

Technically, is metronidazole FDA approved for Giardia treatment in kids?

No (but still an okay answer on the boards if no good alternatives given)

An immigrant child presents with heart block + cardiomyopathy. What ID cause should you consider?

Chagas disease
(American trypanosomiasis)

What are the three main differences between protozoa and helminths (aka "worms")?

Protozoa: Single celled, replicate in human, no eosinophilia

Worms: Multicellular, replicate elsewhere, + eosinophilia

This syndrome of shifting pulmonary infiltrates and eosinophilia can be caused by roundworms. What is the name of the syndrome?

Loffler's syndrome (eosinophilic pneumonia)

A photo of a child living in the southern USA is shown. The foot has a serpiginous line on it. What is the diagnosis?

Hookworm (Necator)

About 1 in 20 people in the USA is infected with which type of roundworm?

Trichinella
(from pork, normally doesn't cause a problem)

The famous "scotch tape test" is used to diagnose what helminthic disorder?

Pinworm
(Enterobius vermicularis)

Pinworms are treated with what medications?

Albendazole/mebendazole

Mnemonic: You need to "bend" to show your itchy butt!

A child from the southern USA with diarrhea, abdominal pain, and rectal prolapse may have what helminth infection?

Whipworm (Trichuria)

Helminths (worms) are not supposed to replicate in the human body. What is the only exception to this rule?

Strongyloides

Does Strongyloides typically cause a noticeable infection?

No – except if the patient becomes immunocompromised –
then they are <u>everywhere!</u>

If Strongyloides causes noticeable infection, what does it cause?
(2 organ systems involved)

Gut – diarrhea
Lungs – cough, pneumonia, & hemorrhagic pneumonia

How is Strongyloides treated?

Ivermectin is the treatment of choice

(thiabendazole was used in the past & was effective, but is no longer made)

Biliary obstruction in someone who has recently visited the Far East & eaten raw fish is probably due to _____?

Clonorchis sinensis
(biliary fluke)

Hematuria results from infection with what fluke?

Schistosoma haematobium

Mnemonic:
Haematobium causes urinary "heme"

Which medication is usually good for killing flukes?

Praziquantel
(decreases "quantity" of flukes!)

Genital herpes is supposed to be due to which herpes simplex virus – 1 or 2?	**2 (usually)**
Facial herpes infections, then, are usually due to which HSV virus?	**HSV 1** (one is on the top, two is on the bottom!)
Asymptomatic shedding of virus is important because _____?	**It allows HSV to spread when no lesions are present** (this is the boards answer – expert opinions vary)
Systemic symptoms are expected with what type of HSV infection?	**Primary –** either type 1 or 2 first time infection
How is acyclovir helpful in a primary herpes infection?	**It shortens the course**
A housekeeper from outside the US starts working in a household here. Soon after, one of the children is brought to the ER with a seizure. Why? *(popular test item!)*	**Cysticercosis in the brain** (eggs in undercooked pork go to brain & retina)
How will you know that a patient has cysticercosis?	**The lesions show up on head CT**
At what point in the worm's life cycle do cysticercosis organisms cause a problem?	**When they die –** **They cause inflammation & seizures**
What is the main treatment for neurocysticercosis?	**Albendazole + steroids (to reduce inflammation)**
A Hispanic child is presented on your boards. He is seizing, and the head CT shows enhancing cystic structures. What is his diagnosis?	**Neurocysticercosis**
If an immunocompromised patient develops primary or recurrent HSV, how should you treat him or her?	**IV acyclovir** *(same for any significantly sick patients suspected to have herpes infections)*

If a pregnant mom has active genital HSV lesions at the time of delivery, what management is recommended?

C-section

(protection from neonatal infection is not complete, but it is helpful)

Serious neonatal HSV infections most often occur in what setting?

Mom acquired an asymptomatic primary HSV 2 infection near time of delivery

If a patient is being admitted to the hospital with a known *Varicella* zoster infection exposure (and the patient is <u>not</u> immune), should the patient be isolated, & if so, for how long?

Yes –

days 8–21 after infection exposure (whether or not the patient has signs of the disease)

(some sources say 10–21)

What type(s) of isolation are needed for Varicella zoster virus (VZV)?

Contact & airborne

(spread in primary infection is mainly via the respiratory system & *very* efficient)

Which patients are most at risk for severe varicella zoster infection & bad complications?
   (3 groups)

- **Immunocompromised (of course)**
- *Adolescents/adults*
- *Pregnant women & preemies/neonates*

For patients at risk of severe Varicella zoster problems, what is the best management if they don't seem to be very ill?

(popular test item!)

Give oral or IV acyclovir, *even if not very ill*

(just prophylactic)

Valacyclovir is also used

If a pregnant adolescent is presented on the boards with varicella zoster infection, what should you do?

(popular test item!)

<u>Give acyclovir</u>

What are the two most common CNS complications of varicella zoster?

(very common on the boards, especially!)

Encephalitis
      &
Transient cerebella ataxia

What is *by far* the most common complication of chicken pox?

(popular test item!)

Staph or strep secondary skin infection

What skin-related complication occurs regularly with chicken pox on the boards?

(2)

(popular test item!)

Toxic shock syndrome

&

Necrotizing fasciitis

If a patient has been given VZIG prophylactically, & is in the hospital, how long will you need to keep the patient in isolation?

28 days!
(days 8–21 only if the patient was exposed but <u>not</u> given VZIG)

Is it alright to immunize a pregnant woman with the varicella vaccine?
(popular test item!)

No

Which chicken pox complication are pregnant patients especially likely to develop?

**Varicella pneumonia
(very bad!)**

Can a pregnant patient be given varicella zoster immunoglobulin?

**Yes –
and <u>should</u> be if she is exposed & seronegative
Acyclovir prophylaxis (7 days) may also be given**

How long can you give varicella zoster IG after exposure?

4 days

Which neonates are at risk for severe varicella zoster infection?

**Those whose moms developed chicken pox in a 7-day window –
5 days before delivery to 2 days after**

(Mom didn't have a chance to make IgG antibodies & transmit them)

If a mom developed chicken pox 6 days before delivery, should you treat the infant as high risk for VZ?

(popular test item!)

<u>No</u>

What should you do for an infant whose mom developed Varicella zoster in the critical 7-day window?

Give VZIG

What is the classic skin finding for infants exposed to varicella zoster in utero?

Cicatricial skin scarring

What is "cicatricial" skin scarring?

Zig-zag scarring on the skin

– with varicella, it often follows a dermatome

(*Cicatricial literally means the type of scar barbed wire would make*)

If a pregnant mom has an outbreak of shingles, is her fetus at risk from the infection?

No

If a mom has a <u>primary</u> varicella zoster infection during pregnancy, when during her pregnancy is the fetus at risk for developing birth defects?

Weeks 8–20

Which patient group at risk for bad Varicella complications should always get acyclovir IV?

The immunocompromised

If a "normal" child develops chicken pox, and is not unusually ill, when would you still consider giving acyclovir?

2nd (or 3rd or 4th) case in one household

Is prednisone used to treat zoster (shingles) in kids?

No
(helpful for adults though)

Is acyclovir useful for the treatment of herpes zoster?

Yes –
decreases lesions & pain

(but probably *not* post-herpetic neuralgia)

CMV causes serious disease in just two settings. What are they?

Immunocompromised
&
Transplacental fetal infection (~1 % of newborns are infected)

What is the most common cause of "blueberry muffin" babies in the USA?

Congenital CMV infection

What is the classic head CT finding for CMV congenital infection babies?

Intracerebral calcifications that circumvent the ventricles
(go around the ventricles)

If mom already has IgG to CMV at the time she becomes pregnant, how does that affect the fetus' chances of developing congenital CMV infection?	**Very unlikely** (<1 %)
Cicatricial skin scarring with limb atrophy sounds like a congenital case of _____?	Varicella zoster
Sensorineural hearing loss and a blueberry muffin baby suggest congenital infection with what organism?	CMV
"Heterophile-negative" mononucleosis-type illness is probably a case of _____ in a normal patient?	CMV
An adolescent patient with HIV presents with vision problems. What is the likely diagnosis?	**CMV retinitis**
There is an important association between bone marrow transplant graft vs. host disease (GCHD) and which infectious diseases?	**CMV** (A donor with antibodies to CMV + a recipient *without* CMV antibodies = increased risk of GVHD)
Does CMV cause infection/inflammation in various organ systems in significantly immunocompromised patients, such as transplant patients?	Yes
If an AIDS patient develops CMV retinitis, what treatment is required?	Valganciclovir *for life* = unless the CD4 count recovers with HAART therapy (then treatment can be discontinued)
In what age group should you <u>not</u> trust the monospot test?	**<4 years old**
How is mononucleosis defined, in terms of labs?	>10 % atypical lymphocytes
Are the majority of EBV infections symptomatic or asymptomatic?	**Asymptomatic**
EBV is associated with what cancer in Africa?	**Burkitt's lymphoma (big mass on jaw)**

EBV is associated with what two types of lymphoma?

Burkitt's

+

B-cell lymphoma

Which EBV serological marker is often positive in patients with Burkitt's that would not be expected in someone long recovered from the primary infection?

EA/R

(EA stands for "early antigen" because antibodies to it appear early in EBV infection)

What sort of *carcinoma* is EBV linked with?

Nasopharyngeal

Is Epstein–Barr virus present for life after the initial infection?

**Yes –
persists in the B-cells**

If a child has a febrile illness, is started on amoxicillin, then develops a rash, what has happened?

(popular test item!)

You have just diagnosed EBV infection

(EBV + amox = rash)

There are several lab tests that are specific for EBV. What does a positive EBNA mean?

The patient is convalescent or done with EBV infection (EBV is Not Active!)

Which lab test tells you that your patient is acutely infected with a primary EBV infection?

(popular test item!)

IgM-VCA

**Mnemonic:
VCA stands for "Very Clearly Acute"**

Which serology is NOT positive with acute, primary, EBV infection?

EBNA (nuclear antigen – not yet making antigens to the deep viral structures in acute phase)

When do EBNA antibodies appear, in the course of EBV infection?

During convalescence

Which antibodies appear first in the acute, primary, EBV infection?

EAs (early antigens) –

Two types are used, named D (diffuse) & R (cytoplasmic)

When does IgM to VCA (viral capsid antigen) appear, relative to when symptoms appear?

About the same time

(IgG production begins shortly after, peaks 2–3 *months* later, then persists at a lower level for life)

In recent EBV infection (past 3–12 months), what serology pattern is expected?

IgG-VCA positive
EBNA positive
EA usually positive

(but no IgM-VCA!)

If a patient has positive EBNA & IgG for VCA, but is EA negative, what is the likely EBV diagnosis?

Long-term (old) EBV infection – >12 months

Which patients sometimes express EA antibodies long term?

Immunocompromised with persistent or frequently reactivating infection

EBV patients will typically have what percentage lymphocytes in the 2nd to 3rd weeks of illness?

>50 %

(about 85 % reach this level of lymphocytosis!)

On peripheral smear, what percentage of lymphocytes should be atypical, to meet EBV laboratory diagnosis criteria?

≥10 %
(most will have 20–40 %)

What sort of cells are the atypicals, generally?

Polyclonal activated CD8 cytotoxic-suppressor T cells

What does the "monospot test" actually test for?

Heterophile antibodies

(it is designed to be a fast test, and just tells you if they are present, not how high the titer of heterophile antibodies is

What is the down side to monospot testing?

Low sensitivity
(around 75 %)

What *are* heterophile antibodies?

A mix of antibodies (polyclonal) produced in response to EBV, but not targeting it.

These antibodies cause agglutination of RBCs from other species, such as horse, sheep, & cows – the tests to identify heterophile antibodies are based on this RBC agglutination

Which patients often do *not* make heterophile antibodies with primary EBV infection?

Young ones <4 years old – & especially common in patients <2 years old

(*about 80% of those <2 years old will not have heterophile antibodies*)

Which serological marker can be used in young patients, to verify primary EBV infection?

EA/R antibodies

(<u>E</u>arly <u>A</u>ntigen R – R is a cytoplasmic antigen)

At what point in the illness are you most likely to get a positive heterophile test?

Weeks 2–3

Starts to decline in weeks 4 & 5

First week is often too early

If a patient is immunocompromised, and you cannot rely on immune-based test results to determine EBV infection, what other lab diagnostic can you use?

PCR for EBV DNA

(can be qualitative or quantitative, depending on what is needed)

EBV is also known as human herpes virus number _____?

Four!

A college student presents with cough, coryza, and conjunctivitis. He is developing a red maculopapular rash. What is it?

Measles!

(*popular test item!*)

Which patients are most likely to present with measles?

Unimmunized <u>or</u> received only one inactivated immunization

(*popular test item!*)

What is the other name for Rubella?

German measles

What are the hallmarks of a German measles infection?

Red rash + lymph nodes in a ring from ear to ear (postauricular-suboccipital LAD)

If a patient is exposed to rubeola/measles, what can you do to prevent infection in an unimmunized patient?

**Immunoglobulin –
you have 6 days to give it**

Measles is most severe in which nutritionally challenged patient population?

(*popular test item!*)

Vitamin A deficient

Koplik spots on the oral mucosa go with which infectious disease?

Measles

Mnemonic: Think of a "*weasel*" in a "*cop's*" uniform *lick*ing a child's cheek to remember that Koplik spots go with measles.

Does rubella also have a special kind of spot?

Yes –
Forchheimer spots
(rose-colored spots on the posterior palate – 1st day only)

(not petechiae)

Which virus causes roseola?

(*popular test item!*)

HHV-6
(human herpes virus-6)

Which virus has recently been shown to be the cause of Kaposi's sarcoma?

(*popular test item!*)

HHV-8
(human herpes virus-8)

What two endocrine disorders are patients with congenital rubella at special risk for developing (oddly enough)?

(*popular test item!*)

IDDM

+

Thyroiditis

(IDDM risk increases 10–20 times)

How does the risk of acquiring congenital rubella infection vary according to the trimester the infection starts?

(*popular test item!*)

It's a "U" – highest in first and third trimester

Although the risk of acquiring a congenital rubella infection is high in both the first and last trimesters, what determines how severe the effects of the infection will be?

(*popular test item!*)

The earlier the infection, the more severe the consequences

What are the usual consequences of   None!
third trimester infection with
congenital rubella?

(*popular test item!*)

Infection with congenital rubella is   Hearing loss or neuro problems
least common in the second trimester.
When it does occur, what general
types of problems usually result?
      (**2 categories**)

(*popular test item!*)

First trimester congenital rubella   Hearing loss & neuro problems
tends to cause what types of problems?
(several systems)   Cataracts & cardiac problems

(*popular test item!*)

Fever, pharyngitis, conjunctivitis,   Pharyngoconjunctival fever
cervical adenitis and rhinitis that   (adenovirus 3)
affects a whole group of summer camp
kids who've been swimming is
_____?

Adenovirus most commonly causes   Gut – diarrhea
URI, but what other body systems   (types 40 & 41)
does it sometimes affect?
      (**2**)   Bladder – hemorrhagic
       Cystitis (types 11 & 21)

Summer, swimming and group   Adenovirus 3 (pharyngoconjunctival
outbreaks of URI are associated with   fever)
which virus?

If the boards presents an epidemic   SARS (severe acute respiratory
serious respiratory disease, and the   syndrome)
cause is identified as a coronavirus,
what is the diagnosis?

What kind of inflammatory process does   Interstitial pneumonitis
RSV cause in the lung?

If a child requires prophylaxis for   RSV antibodies
RSV, what is given?

(*popular test item!*)

Should ribavirin be used with RSV infection?

No –
Recent studies showed no effect

What sort of infection does parainfluenza virus usually cause?

Same as RSV, but occurs all year

Which types of influenza are the main causes for concern?

A + B

Amantadine/rimantadine are mainly effective against which sorts of influenza?

Type A

Mnemonic:
A is for Amantadine

What is the best way to prevent influenza infection?

Immunize!

Is immunization against influenza recommended for children <9 years old?

Yes

(*popular test item!*)

What is the influenza immunization schedule for kids <9 years?

2 shots, 1 month apart

The newer neuraminidase anti-influenza drugs are effective against which influenza types(s)?

Both A + B

(but they're not wildly effective – best when used early in the infection)

For which age groups are the two neuraminidase anti-influenza drugs recommended?
(different for each drug)

Oseltamivir (Tamiflu®) –
treatment from 14 days old
prophylaxis from 3 months old

Zanamivir(Relenza®) –
treatment from 7 years old
prophylaxis from 5 years old

What contraindication to the use of zanamivir (Relenza®) should you screen for?

Allergy to milk protein

On the board exam, which infectious agent causes hand–foot–mouth disease?

Coxsackie virus
(can also be enterovirus, but not usually)

In infants, hand–foot–mouth disease also sometimes affects what part of the body?

Diaper area

What happens in hand–foot–mouth disease?	**– Rash, sometimes with vesicles, on hands & feet** **– Vesicles on lips, tongue, gums, buccal mucosa**
The board is especially fond of presenting hand–foot–mouth disease in what format?	**Photo section!**
If a patient is presented with myocarditis or pericarditis, and the patient is from the USA, what is the likely cause? (infectious agent	**Coxsackie virus**
Acute hemorrhagic conjunctivitis gives your patient some scary looking eyes. What usually causes it? (2 viruses)	Enterovirus (#70) & Coxsackie virus (type A24)
What infectious agent causes herpangina?	Coxsackie A (*not herpes*)
What does herpangina look like?	**Little vesicles on pharynx, tonsils, uvula**
Why is herpangina a problem in pediatrics?	**Hydration – the throat gets very sore & they won't drink**
If you are asked to differentiate herpangina from herpes, what is the main differentiator?	**Herpangina causes a sore throat – Herpes usually cause skin/labial sores**
Why should you avoid treating Salmonella with antibiotics, unless it is medically necessary?	Increases likelihood of carrier state
What is the best possible specimen to give you the best chance of identifying TB infection, if it is present?	**Early morning gastric aspirate**
If a child's fever resolves suddenly, and a red spotted rash appears equally suddenly, what is the infection?	**Roseola** (human herpes virus 6 – HHV6)
Which infection sometimes causes Pastia's lines, and what are they?	Scarlet fever – increased erythema in the creases of flexor surfaces

An immigrant child from Haiti presents with an asymmetric flaccid paralysis, loss of DTRs, and a fever. What is the disorder?	**Polio**
Does the paralysis that accompanies polio develop slowly or rapidly?	**Rapid – It is maximal within 4 days**
To qualify as a case of polio, there must be neurological deficits after what length of time?	**60 days**
If a human is infected with rabies, will he/she develop hydrophobia (fear of water) like animals do?	**Yes – perceiving food or water causes larynx/pharynx spasms – that's why infected animals/humans fear them**
How is rabies definitively diagnosed?	**Nerve biopsy from the "nape of neck" (back of neck) shows "Negri bodies"**
What is the risk of rabies from bites of fox, skunk or bats in the USA?	**High – assume they're rabid** (unless you catch them and check their brains)
Do ferrets carry rabies?	**Yes**
If a domestic pet is not rabies immunized, and it bites someone, does the person need all of the rabies shots?	**No – observe the animal for 10 days – if it remains well it doesn't have rabies** (*The exception is a high-risk bite to face or neck – start immunizations!*)
Do rodents or rabbits carry rabies?	**No**
If rabies prophylaxis is indicated, what do you give?	**IgG & vaccine** (IgG is given once, vaccine is a series)
Is it alright to give rabies IgG and rabies vaccine at the same site on the body? (*popular test item!*)	**No! That would be silly because they'll just bind to each other & not do your patient any good!**
On the boards, if an adolescent male gets mumps, what complication will he develop?	**Orchitis**

On the boards if an adolescent *female* gets mumps, what complication will she develop?

Oophoritis or mastitis

Is the oophoritis that sometimes occurs with mumps likely to cause female infertility?

No
(in reality, orchitis rarely does either)

Parotid gland swelling, either unilateral or bilateral, should make you think of what three possible etiologies?

1. **Mumps (uni or bilateral)**
2. **Parotitis (usually unilateral)**
3. **Bulimia**

Mumps commonly affects which organ systems?

Parotid gland
Gonads
CNS (deafness sometimes)

Polio infection is usually accompanied by what sort of typical CNS infection signs?

Meningitis signs

(It's aseptic, if you do the tap)

What are the two patterns of paralysis in polio paralytic disease?

Spinal – proximal strength most affected

Bulbar – swallowing, respiration, & brain-stem affected

What is the reservoir for Hantavirus infection?

Rodents

Why is Babesiosis associated with the "maltese cross" buzzword?

Because there are usually multiple organisms in the cell, & sometimes they arrange themselves like a cross

What causes 5th Disease?

Parvovirus B19

With 5th Disease (erythema infectiosum), is it alright for the child to return to school if they have the rash?

Yes –
When the rash appears they are no longer infectious!

How do you make the diagnosis of parvovirus B19 infection, based on labs?

IgM (or IgG) to the virus, or PCR

(most cases are diagnosed clinically)

How does parvovirus B19 affect a fetus if the mom contracts the infection during pregnancy?

Usually no effect –
5–10 % fetal loss

If a parent or grandparent presents with polyarthritis, especially of finger joins, +/− a rash, what are they trying to tell you the child had/has?

Parvovirus B19

An adolescent from the South western USA presents with a pneumonia that develops after a flu-like illness. It sounds like Staph pneumonia superinfection, except that the vignette includes the hematocrit (high), platelets (low), and albumin (low). What is it?

Hantavirus

How is HIV most commonly transmitted in the developing world, and often in the US, as well?

Heterosexual contact

When did the USA begin effective HIV screening of the blood supply?

1985

When does most vertical HIV (mother to infant) transmission occur?

Labor & delivery

Is it alright for HIV+ moms to breast feed?

No

How is spread of HIV to health care workers prevented?

Universal precautions

In a boards vignette, you are given a patient who has just been diagnosed with TB. What other test would you like to do?
(*popular test item!*)

HIV screening!

A sickle cell patient develops an aplastic crisis. What virus is likely to be responsible?

Parvovirus B19

Are hemophiliacs in the pediatric population likely to be HIV infected?

**No −
The blood supply was effectively screened beginning in 1985 & recombinant factors are now used**

At what age can standard screening tests for HIV be used?

18 months

What are the standard screening tests for HIV?

ELISA, then if positive confirm with Western blot

Mnemonic:
Think of "Elisa" as the receptionist—
she does the initial screening

In children 0–18 months old, how can you check for HIV infection?

PCR testing for HIV DNA or RNA

(96 % sensitive & 99 % specific at 1 month old)

If an infant may be HIV infected, when should you attempt to check for HIV status?

Repeatedly –
1st in first 48 h of life
2nd attempt at 1 month
3rd attempt at 3–6 months

(some recommend an additional attempt at day 14, to identify more infants earlier)

If the possibly HIV infected infant has a positive PCR test, what should you do?

Repeat the PCR –
Two are required to confirm the diagnosis

What do you need to confirm that the infant is *not* HIV infected?

Requires two negative HIV PCRs, at least 1 month apart, in an infant 6 months of age or older

OR

At least two negative PCR results in an infant 4 months or older, who is not breast feeding (first test must be from after 1 month old)

Infants of HIV positive mothers should also be serologically screened for what additional disorders?
(3)

Hep C (along with Hep B, of course)

Syphilis

Toxoplasmosis

A child is referred to you because HIV screening has come up positive. Mom is known to have HIV. The child is 6 months old. What do you want to know about the testing?

Whether the PCR test was done

(The ELISA & Western blot rely on IgG, which is always positive in infants of infected moms due to transplacental IgG transfer)

Hantavirus patients will often have a full recovery, if proper supportive care is provided. What are the two problems that put Hanta patients at risk of dying?	**Pulmonary edema** & **Impaired cardiac function**
How likely is an HIV infected mom to pass her virus to her infant during pregnancy and delivery, if she does not take antiretroviral medications?	20–30 % chance
If an HIV positive mom takes antiretroviral medications during pregnancy, can she significantly lower the probability of vertical transmission to her infant?	**Yes – to a few percent!!!**
What two feeding practices must HIV positive mothers be warned against, to reduce chances of postnatal HIV transmission?	**Breast feeding (assuming safe infant formula available)** & **Premastication (chewing food *for* the baby) – proven transmission link!**
If an infant has frequent candidal infections, or persistent lymphadenopathy or HSM (hepatosplenomegaly), what diagnosis should you consider?	**HIV infection**
Parotitis in the first year of life is unusual and should make you consider _____?	**HIV infection**
At what CD4 count should patients be considered severely immuno-compromised?	**<200**
Are there situations in which a CD4 count greater than the usual cutoff should be used to designate severe immunocompromise/AIDS?	**Yes – young children** **<12 months = <750 CD4s** **1–5 years old = <500 CD4s**

In addition to tuberculosis, what other disease presentations in adolescents should make you consider HIV infection?	**1. ITP** **2. Serious bacterial pneumonia** **3. Recurrent zoster**
What is the most common opportunistic infection for HIV patients? (*popular test item!*)	*P. carinii* (*now renamed P. jiroveci! but the disorder is still called "PCP"*)
What are the two best medications for treatment of *P. jiroveci* (formerly *P. carinii*)?	**TMP/SMX** **Or** **IV Pentamidine** (aerosol is used for prophylaxis, not treatment)
When is prednisone indicated as part of the treatment for pneumocystis?	**Pa O$_2$<70 mmHg**
Should neonates or very young infants who <u>may</u> have HIV be prophylaxed for PCP? (*P. jiroveci*) (*popular test item!*)	**Yes!**
If an infant is HIV positive, or the HIV status is still unclear, what is appropriate PCP prophylaxis?	**Give TMP/SMX until confirmed HIV negative** **Or** **Until 12 month old if HIV positive (reassess regimen at 12 months)**
At what age should you start PCP prophylaxis?	Most sources recommend 6 weeks
Should infants at risk for HIV infection be started on treatment before the HIV infection is confirmed?	Yes! Start zidovudine as soon as possible after birth! Begin cART (combined antiretroviral therapy) when the infant is older, even if initial testing is negative

By what age should an infant begin on a combination HIV treatment regimen?

Current research indicates beginning *before 12 weeks* of age provides important health & developmental benefits!

(In some cases, cART is started much earlier, but safety & outcome data is limited. Functional "HIV cure" has been reported in one child whose cART was begun at 30 h)

After the age of 1 year, what should guide your decision as to whether PCP prophylaxis is needed or not?

CD4 criteria for severe immunosuppression
(<500 aged 1 thru 5 years)
(<200 older than 5 years)

*The children aged 1–5 years must keep their count **at or above 500 for 3 months** to discontinue prophylaxis*

If your patient needs TMP/SMX prophylaxis for PCP, but can't tolerate it, what alternative medication can be used?

Dapsone – check for G6PD deficiency <u>before</u> you use!

Atovaquone is also an option

What is a "banana gametocyte" on a blood smear, and what does it signify?

- **An RBC elongated like a banana, due to malaria parasite(s) in it!**
- **Usually *P. falciparum***

If you give dapsone, you must first check for what condition?

G6PD deficiency

Which children can use pentamidine for PCP prophylaxis?

Only those older than 5 – It is aerosolized & must be used properly

If you are evaluating an HIV positive patient for TB, and the PPD is negative, how should you interpret this?

Encouraging, but not definitive – Patient may be anergic (non-reactive)

MAC/MAI are opportunistic lung infections. When might a pediatric patient need prophylaxis for them, and what do you give?

- **Severe immunocompromise**
- **Give azithromycin or clarithromycin**

What two recurrent types of candidal infections do the boards like to present *to suggest HIV infection*?

Thrush

&

Diaper rash (dermatitis)

Molluscum contagiosum – what does it look like?

**Small papules/vesicles with umbilicated centers (dot in the center) –
Not red**

A lot of difficulty with molluscum contagiosum should make you think about _____?

Possible HIV infection

Bad diarrhea can develop with isospora infection in the immunocompromised. How is it treated?

TMP/SMX

Cryptosporidium tends to cause a severe and chronic diarrhea in the immuno-compromised. How is it treated?

Nitazoxanide is first line

(Paromomycin with azithromycin is another option, but much less effective in clearing the parasites)

What should patients recovering from cryptosporidium be instructed NOT to do, in terms of activities?

NO Swimming until 2 weeks after symptom resolution –
Crypto now causes more than 50 % of all US public swimming pool-related outbreaks

What unusual attribute of cryptosporidium allows it to be so successful with swimmers?

It is not affected by chlorine!

What is the treatment for toxoplasmosis when it activates and affects the eyes or CNS?

**Pyrimethamine +
Leucovorin +
Sulfadiazine**

**Mnemonic:
PLS help me to see!**

Steroids are also sometimes given

When the toxoplasmosis treatment regimen is started, what medication must be included to protect the hematologic system?

(popular test item!)

**Folinic acid
(the active form of folate –
folic acid will not work)**

FOLINIC ACID=LEUCOVORIN
(same thing)

Extended use of pyrimethamine should always be combined with what supplement?	**Folinic acid** (to prevent anemia)
If a health care worker has been exposed to meningococcus, does he/she need chemoprophylaxis?	**Only if exposure to droplets was likely** (e.g., intubation, mouth-to-mouth) *Pay attention – This is a change!*
Aside from the CD4 count, how do you know when you should start antiretroviral therapy? (3 ways)	**Symptoms – The patient becomes symptomatic** (AIDS defining illness or significant symptoms) **Age – infant < 12 months old** **RNA level – >100,000 plasma HIV RNA level**
The side effect most associated with AZT is _____?	**Anemia/pancytopenia**
Which reverse transcriptase inhibitors tend to cause pancreatitis and peripheral neuropathy (painful)?	**ddI + ddC** **Mnemonic: The "D's" go with the "P's,"** (as in "poopy diaper!")
Abacavir is a type of reverse transcriptase inhibitor. What is it most important to know about this med?	**The hypersensitivity reaction consists of a flu-like illness and rash – giving the med again after this reaction = <u>death</u>** **Mnemonic: Sudden death will take you "aback"** (shock you)!
How can you prevent the abacavir reaction?	**It occurs *only* in patients with a particular HLA type: HLA-B*5701 – screen for the HLA type before starting the med**
Which patients are most likely to develop the abacavir reaction?	**European descent** (about 5 % carry the HLA-B*5701 type)
Efavirenz is an NNRTI med (non-nucleoside reverse transcriptase inhibitor). What is it most important to know about this med?	**TERATOGENIC**

An adolescent HIV patient presents with kidney stones. What med is he taking?

Crixivan®
(Indinavir)

A boards vignette tells you that your patient has just reached the point with HIV where antiretrovirals need to be started. Should you start treatment with a single drug or multiple drugs?

Multidrug "cART" – Stands for "combination AntiRetroviral Therapy"

(sometimes abbreviated ARV for AntiRetroViral therapy)

(start with three)

(*In the USA, testing for resistance is recommended*)

How do you know which combinations of antiretrovirals are UNacceptable?
(2 rules)

1. don't choose an answer with ddC in the choices
2. any answer with ZDV/D4T is wrong!

All cART regimens include a "dual" nucleoside/nucleotide reverse transcriptase inhibitor, a two-drug combination referred to as the "backbone." Which combination is acceptable for children in any age group?

Zidovudine

+

Lamivudine or Emtricitabine

At what age may abacavir replace zidovudine?

3 months or older
(remember to check HLA type before beginning abacavir)

Tenofovir can replace zidovudine or abacavir in the adolescent cART regimen. What additional benefit does tenofovir have, in terms of antiviral efficacy?

It is also effective against hepatitis B (for those patients with both)

In addition to tenofovir, which other cART medications have activity against hepatitis B?

Emtricitabine & lamivudine

In HIV, it is best to have a level of viremia so low that you can't detect it. At what level is the viremia considered to be really high?

>50,000 copies (per mL)

When should you switch drug regimens for HIV suppression?
(3 situations)

Drug toxicity

Clinical worsening

Significant worsening in labs (meaning viral load climbing or not suppressed by treatment)

The CDC defines three levels of HIV infection. What are they, & what defines each level?

Levels A, B, & C –
A – Asymptomatic & no history of symptoms

B – Symptoms attributable to T cell dysfunction or HIV itself, or symptoms that were complicated by HIV infection

C – AIDS-defining opportunistic infections have occurred

A nurse spilled urine from an HIV patient onto her skin. She had some scratches on her skin. Should she take post-exposure prophylaxis?

(popular test item!)

<u>No</u> (urine doesn't count)

If a health care worker is exposed to bloody fluid, and the skin exposed was <u>not</u> completely intact, should the healthcare worker take post-exposure prophylaxis?

(popular test item!)

Yes

What is the main antiretroviral given to pregnant women?

Zidovudine

How should antiretroviral medication be given during labor and delivery (PO, IM, IV, PR)?

IV

Which medication, if any, should newborns at risk for HIV be given?

Zidovudine
(until 6 weeks of age)

**Mnemonic:
Makes sense – it's what their moms are likely to be taking!**

In what circumstances will you need to give newborn HIV prophylactic treatment with two different drugs?	**If the mother has NOT been taking combination antiretroviral therapy – Baby must then receive 6 weeks of zidovudine** **+** **3 doses of nevirapine in the first week of life**
How long should the newborn remain on the HIV medication regimen?	**6 weeks** *– start within 6–12 h of birth, if possible*
Should premature infants at risk for HIV also be started on a prophylactic medication regimen?	**Yes, the same regimen as for term infants**
Should infants with HIV be started on the same immunization schedule as other infants?	**Yes –** **Modify only for live vaccines, if severe immunocompromise is present**
If a pregnant mom is diagnosed as HIV positive during her pregnancy, how should her preventative plan be different from a non-pregnant HIV positive mom?	**No different –** **Except avoid teratogens efavirenz & ddI/d4T**
What is the best predictor of long-term outcome in HIV, for a patient who is still early on in the disease process? *(popular test item!)*	**Viral load**
What is HAART? (used in HIV treatment)	**<u>H</u>ighly <u>A</u>ctive <u>A</u>nti-<u>R</u>etroviral <u>T</u>herapy** (combination therapy utilizing drugs with six different types of mechanisms to limit the virus's success as much as possible!)
Kaposi's lesions may occasionally be seen in adolescents with HIV. What causes Kaposi's?	**HHV-8** **(Human Herpes Virus #8)**

An adolescent presents with a flu-like syndrome with pharyngitis and rash. The question mentions that the adolescent is sexually active. What should you investigate?

(*popular test item!*)

HIV –
could be "acute retroviral syndrome."
(occurs 2–4 weeks after initial infection)

What is the main use for <u>inhaled</u> pentamidine?

<u>Prophylaxis</u> for PCP in those >5 years old

(for <u>treatment</u>, use IV)

An HIV positive patient is being treated for a bad case of PCP, and begins to seize. What should you suspect?

Hypoglycemia – (bizarre side effect of pentamidine – it destroys islet cells → either high or low glucose)

How does HIV infection affect CNS development in very young children?

The majority have some level of encephalopathy (directly caused by HIV)

What has the impact of HAART been on CNS effects of HIV in the very young?

It prevents or slows it

(<u>h</u>ighly <u>a</u>ctive <u>a</u>nti-<u>r</u>etroviral <u>t</u>herapy)

A patient from El Salvador, HIV positive, with pneumonia, palatal ulcers, splenomegaly, and bone-marrow suppression = what diagnosis?

Histoplasmosis

If a patient is started on PCP prophylaxis, when is it alright to <u>stop</u> prophylaxis?

CD4 count >200 for more than 3 months, following initiation of HAART regimen

What is the gold standard for diagnosing PCP?

Silver staining of samples from bronchoscopy or bronchoalveolar lavage

Are there indications for stopping MAC/MAI prophylaxis in an HIV patient, *if the patient actually had the infection*?

Controversial –
For the boards, <u>no</u>, do not stop prophylaxis

What is the most common cause of cardiac death due to endocarditis infection?

CHF

If valve dysfunction is significant enough to harm ventricular function in a patient with SBE, what is recommended?	Surgical correction (Conduction deficit is also a reason for surgery)
What is the most important test for diagnosing endocarditis?	Blood cultures
What two organisms most commonly cause endocarditis in children?	**#1 Strep viridans** & **#2 Staph aureus**
When doing a bacteremia work-up, which children should definitely get a urine culture?	Boys <6 months, Girls <12 months
What is the most common pathogen for UTIs in very young infants (less than 2 months old)?	E. coli
Bacterial gastroenteritis is not very common in infants <2 months old. When it happens, what is the likely bacterium?	Salmonella
What are the most common causes of bacteremia in infants, birth to 2 months old?	Group B Strep & *E. coli* (Listeria is not as common but must be covered)
Patients with surgical valves (prosthetic valves) are most likely to develop endocarditis due to what organism?	Staph epidermidis
If a patient has endocarditis, he or she nearly always has what other problem?	Either congenital or rheumatic heart problems (or a history of instrumentation)
If a patient clinically appears to have endocarditis, but no organisms are detected on blood culture, what causes should you suspect?	**HACEK** **(Haemophilus Actinobacillus** **Cardiobacterium** **Eikenella** **Kingella)**

Why are HACEK organisms so tough to culture?

They're "fastidious" Gram negatives, and take >7 days to grow!

In addition to HACEK organisms, are there any other causes of culture negative endocarditis you should know about?

Fungus
Q fever (*Coxiella burnetii*)
Legionella
Chlamydia

What are Janeway spots, and what do they indicate?

• non-tender spots on hands and feet
• acute bacterial endocarditis

Where are Roth spots found, and what do they signify?

• white spots on the retina
• subacute bacterial endocarditis (they develop late in the course)

The three famous signs associated with endocarditis are: _____ _____ & _____?

Roth spots
Janeway lesions

&

Osler nodes (usually subacute endocarditis)

Which of the famous signs of bacterial endocarditis is/are painful?

Only Osler nodes
Mnemonic: Remember "only Osler offends," or think about how painful it can be to write up a good Oslerian H&P!

If a patient with perfectly normal valves develops endocarditis, what is the likely pathogen?

Staph aureus

Overall, the most common pathogen to cause endocarditis in the pediatric population is _____?

Strep viridans
(usually in hearts with congenital or rheumatic problems)

What is the recommended treatment for this most common pediatric endocarditis pathogen?

Penicillin G

Or

Ceftriaxone

(other regimens are also possible)

Endocarditis + prosthetic valve usually = what kind of treatment?

Surgical

(The exception is *S. epidermidis* with subacute presentation)

Is vancomycin a preferred medication for treatment of endocarditis?	No – It is used when necessary (due to PCN allergy or methicillin resistant species), but it is overall less effective
If a HACEK organism causes endocarditis, what is the recommended treatment regimen?	Ceftriaxone Or Ampicillin with gentamicin
Most other causes of pediatric endocarditis can be treated with which two antibiotic regimens?	Ampicillin & gentamicin Or Penicillin G (high doses required for resistant organisms)
How long is the treatment regimen for endocarditis?	Generally 4 weeks
Should you wait to get CSF cultures before starting antibiotics in suspected bacterial meningitis?	**No!** (The CSF is still good for culture for a while after antibiotics are started, and you can't take chances with meningitis!)
For AIDS patients, or others with severe immunocompromise, be sure to ask for what unusual lab evaluation of CSF, if meningitis is suspected?	India ink or cryptococcal antigen (both for possible *cryptococcus*)
If a boards vignette tells you that your CSF tap has "what appear to be white cells swimming in it," what is the diagnosis? (*popular test item!*)	**<u>Amebic</u> meningitis (yuck!)**
Swimming in a cow pond or "brackish" water is associated with what type of meningitis? (*popular test item!*)	**<u>Amebic</u>** **(Nigleria is the organism)**
Encephalitis that results in death is usually due to what pathogen?	Herpes simplex
What is the most common general cause of encephalitis (for those cases that have an identified cause)?	Arboviruses (St. Louis, Eastern equine, West Nile, etc.)

Diarrhea occurring with antibiotic use is usually due to _____?	A side effect due to change in gut flora
Colitis following antibiotic use is often due to _____?	*C. difficile* (assay for *C. diff* cytotoxin in stool)
History of seafood ingestion or exposure to the Gulf of Mexico + liver failure = infection with what organism? (*popular test item!*)	***Vibrio vulnificus*** (also causes skin lesions)
Shellfish diarrhea is often the work of which bacterial family?	**Vibrio's**
If you need to work up a patient with diarrhea, what stool studies should you send?	Fecal WBCs Stool C&S O&P
Diarrheal outbreaks on cruise ships are usually due to which pathogen? (*popular test item!*)	**Noroviruses** (*formerly called Norwalk-type viruses*)
When should you definitely avoid antimotility agents with diarrhea patients?	**Bloody diarrhea or positive fecal WBCs**
What non-infectious cause of diarrhea also causes WBCs to end up in the stool?	**IBD** (Inflammatory Bowel Disease)
Noroviruses (Norwalk-type viruses) are also associated with what food products? (2 categories)	Clams & oysters Leafy greens
In an adolescent or young woman, is pyuria alone enough to treat for UTI?	Yes (no C&S needed)
For which patient groups is it alright to treat for UTI, if all they have is asymptomatic bacteremia?	**Pregnant** **Diabetic** **Transplant/neutropenic**
What organisms are commonly found in brain abscesses?	Pneumococcus H. flu Anaerobes (usually coming from nearby infections like sinusitis)

What are the four most common causes of diarrhea in US children?	Norovirus is the main cause (especially in children ≤18 months old)
	Rotavirus (dropping due to vaccination)
	Adenoviruses (types 40 & 41 mainly)
	Astroviruses
What are the top four causes of childhood diarrhea in the world?	Rotavirus
	Shigella
	Cryptosporidium
	ST-ETEC (Toxigenic *E. coli* with Shiga toxin)
How long should you treat an uncomplicated UTI in a child or adolescent?	3–5 days (TMP/SMX preferred, nitrofurantoin or amoxicillin/clavulanate also good options)
Which aspect of a child's history can give you a clue as to whether he or she is likely to have an antibiotic resistant UTI?	History of prior antibiotic use (e.g., for otitis media) – Kids with frequent prior antibiotic use are more likely to develop UTIs resistant to those antibiotics
Is ciprofloxacin alright as a second-line therapy for UTI in children?	Yes – the CDC approved it for kids ages 1–17 with UTI in 2004
Which organism is associated with renal stones when it causes UTIs?	Proteus (a "urea-splitting organism")
If a pregnant patient develops pyelonephritis, what is the correct management?	Admit for IV antibiotics (cephalosporins, ampicillin, aminoglycosides are okay)
Can children with pyelonephritis be treated as outpatients?	Yes – IF The patient is nontoxic appearing & the UTI is uncomplicated (no stones, etc.)
	There is a reliable & competent caregiver
	Able to follow-up in 24 h
	Car & telephone available
	The patient can take PO & has no need of hospital-based medical support

What is the story with Bactrim® (TMP/SMX) in pregnancy?

Linked to kernicterus in <u>late</u> pregnancy and in young infants who are breastfeeding

Which organism is the "fishtank bacillus?"

M. marinum
(*Mycobacterium marinum*)

Large hemorrhagic bullae, plus other skin lesions that look like an "angry volcano," are associated with which Vibrio species?

Vulnificus!

Mnemonic:
Sounds like "volcano"

If a vignette sounds like it's supposed to be osteomyelitis, but an X-ray of the area provides no evidence for osteomyelitis, what should you assume?

(popular test item!)

It's still probably osteomyelitis

(it takes 10–14 days for changes to appear on x-ray)

What is the earliest sign of osteomyelitis on x-ray?

(popular test item!)

"periosteal elevation"

(inflammation lifts the periosteum up from the bone enough to be seen separately)

If you suspect osteomyelitis, but a (pyrophosphate) bone scan is negative, what should you assume?

A negative bone scan rules out osteomyelitis

If you suspect osteomyelitis, and obtain a positive bone scan, what should you assume?

Nothing –
Positive bone scan supports osteomyelitis <u>but</u> can also indicate malignancy, fracture, etc.

Which other radiological study is also highly sensitive for detecting osteomyelitis, but more specific than a bone scan?

MRI –
Also shows soft tissue & joint complications

How should you identify the causative organism in osteomyelitis?

Bone biopsy/scraping or fluid for culture & Gram stain

If an osteomyelitis is draining pus through a fistula, can you use a culture and sensitivity of the fluid to identify the organism?

(popular test item!)

No –
Oddly enough, it will not consistently grow out the correct (causative) organism

Osteomyelitis – IVDA – pelvic or veterbral sites = what organism?

Pseudomonas

(or possibly Staph aureus)

Menstruating adolescent – sexually active – fever – joint paint = what disorder?

Gonorrhea septic arthritis

Septic arthritis is most common in which patient group?

Kids <3 years old

How is septic arthritis treated?
   (two components)

- Drain infected joint fluid
- IV Abx for 6 weeks

(open drainage in OR sometimes performed)

An epidemic of any illness among patients in the hospital is usually due to?

Spread via the worker's <u>hands</u>

If a patient develops a line infection, we ordinarily pull the line, culture the catheter (tip), and give antibiotics. In what situations may the line be left in place while antibiotics are given to clear the infection?

When the line is essential to patient care & cannot easily be replaced – this is called "salvage" of the catheter

If "line salvage" is attempted, what is special about the way the antibiotics are administered?

They must be given via the "antibiotic lock technique" – if that is not possible, then the antibiotics must be administered through the catheter suspected to be infected

What is the antibiotic lock technique, in general terms?

High concentrations of an appropriate antibiotic are instilled directly into the lumen of the infected catheter

(heparin may or may not be used along with the antibiotic)

If line salvage is attempted, how do you know whether it is successful or not?

Obtain blood cultures after 72 h of antibiotics effective for the infecting organism have been given – if two sets of cultures are positive, the line needs to be removed

Note: one set of positive cultures is enough in a neonate

How do quinolones interrupt bacterial multiplication?

Disrupt function of DNA gyrase (DNA cannot be put back after it is used for protein synthesis)

Which antibiotics block ribosomal subunits, preventing the bacteria from producing proteins?

Macrolides, Oxazolidinones, Aminoglycosides and Tetracyclines

Mnemonic:
MOAT – Think of antibiotics forming a MOAT around the body blocking disease

AT 30, antibiotics stop disease, at 50, you need MO' (more). This mnemonic is supposed to help you remember which antibiotic classes act on the 30s and 50s ribosomal units. How does it work?

AT 30: <u>A</u>minoglycosides and <u>T</u>etracyclines bind the 30s unit

At 50, MO: <u>M</u>acrolides and <u>O</u>xazolidinones (linezolid) bind the 50s

What treatment protocol is essential to decreasing the risk of HIV transmission from mothers to infants?

**IV Zidovudine during labor/delivery
&
Zidovudine after birth (PO) for the infant**

Which HIV infected mothers may *not* need IV zidovudine during labor & delivery?

Those on cART with viral RNA levels consistently ≤1,000, and good continued adherence to the cART regimen at time of delivery

Should the babies of these mothers still receive zidovudine after birth?

**Yes –
But only zidovudine
(nevirapine is not required)**

Is an elective c-section helpful in reducing HIV transmission?

**Yes, *at 38 weeks* (to avoid spontaneous delivery) *if* the mother's viral RNA level is >1,000
(for mothers with low viral RNA levels, benefit is unclear)**

If an infant born to an HIV positive mother presents with severe neurological findings, or is otherwise severely ill without explanation, what HIV-related cause should you consider?

Mitochondrial dysfunction due to exposure to cART medications (NRTIs, in particular)

At what point should pneumocystis pneumonia prophylaxis be started in a possibly HIV-positive infant?

When the zidovudine regimen has been completed

(generally around 6 weeks – some infants may receive just 4 weeks of zidovudine is the mother's viral load was very well controlled)

What hematological test should routinely be obtained on infants born to mothers on cART & zidovudine?

CBC for hematological abnormalities

What is the *main way* to diagnose endocarditis?

(*popular test item!*)

Blood cultures

How do you know whether a head CT is required before doing an LP for possible meningitis?

Focal neurological findings = CT *otherwise you don't need it*

(*and shouldn't get it! Delay in care!*)

How is chronic meningitis defined?

Slow onset with symptoms evolving over >7 days

If a meningitis patient has focal findings and therefore needs a head CT before you can LP, what do you do?

(3 steps)

1. **Start antibiotics**
2. **Get the head CT**
3. **LP if there isn't a mass**

What are the components of the blood–brain barrier?

(*popular test item!*)

1. **Arachnoid membrane**
2. **Choroid plexus epithelium**
3. **Endothelia of the cerebral micro-vasculature**

Which of the three portions of the blood–brain barrier is most likely to be breached (leak)?

(*popular test item!*)

Choroid plexus
(unless there was trauma, of course)

If a vignette mentions that the patient has had multiple bouts of meningitis, and has a past history of head trauma, what are they trying to tell you?

There is an intracranial communication with something like a sinus, due to the old trauma

If a patient is specifically described as having repeated bouts of meningitis due to _N. meningitidis_, what should you suspect?

(_popular test item!_)

A complement deficiency

How do you test for complement deficiency?

CH50 or CH100
(tests the classic hemolytic pathway for 50 % or 100 % lysis of sheep RBCs)

&

AP50
(testing the alternative pathway)

A boards vignette tells you that your patient has _N. meningitis_. It asks, "what else do you want to look for?"

(_popular test item!_)

Complement deficiency
(terminal complement deficiency)

Which organisms are splenectomized patients at special risk to develop?
(general category,
and three specific ones)

– **Encapsulated organisms**
– _**S. pneumo**_
– _**H. flu**_
– _**N. meningitidis**_

Splenectomized patients are also at special risk to develop bad infection from which parasitic disorders?

Babesiosis & malaria

Why should a splenectomized patient be especially worried after a dog bite?

More susceptible to serious Capnocytophagia

Aseptic meningitis means the same thing as _____ meningitis?

Non-bacterial
(almost always viral)

What do you expect to see in the CSF of a patient with bacterial meningitis?

↑ **neutrophils**
↑ **protein**
↓ **glucose**

What do you expect to see in the CSF of a patient with TB meningits?

Basically very similar to bacterial, except more monocytes than neutrophils

Syphilis can occasionally produce meningitis. What will the CSF show?	**Low everything-** **WBCs – a few** **Glucose – low** **Protein – low**
In aseptic meningitis, what should the CSF profile look like? *(popular test item!)*	**Some WBCs – more lymphs than PMNs** **Glucose – nl** **Protein – nl**
If a vignette mentions that an LP was done, and there was a predominance of PMNs, but that the LP was repeated a little later and showed mainly lymphocytes, what are they trying to tell you? *(popular test item!)*	**It's viral – PMNs still predominate very early (but of course, no bacteria will be seen)**
Peds boards sometimes give you a table of antibiotic susceptibilities, or the same information in the vignette. What number indicates that the organism is definitely susceptible to a particular antibiotic? *(popular test item!)*	**≤0.5** (μg/ml)
If you are treating a meningitis patient with Strep pneumo, and the sensitivity comes back at 1.0-2.0 for ceftriaxone, what should you do?	<u>Continue</u> ceftriaxone & **Add vancomycin**
If your pneumococcal meningitis patient has bacteria sensitive to ceftriaxone, but you have already started him or her on ceftriaxone + vancomycin, what should you do?	**Stop the <u>vanc</u>** (continue with ceftriaxone only)
If a sensitivity comes back in the 1.0 – 2.0 μg/ml area, how should you interpret it?	**The organism is *resistant – but multidrug therapy may still work***
In general, on the boards, what is the guiding principle in antibiotic selection?	**The simplest, oldest, least sophisticated agent that will kill the bug is preferred**

Gram positive diplococci = what organism? *(usually)* *(popular test item!)*	**Pneumococcus**
Gram positive rods = what organism? *(popular test item!)*	**Listeria** **(ampicillin kills it)**
Gram-negative rods are usually which organism? *(popular test item!)*	*E. coli*
Pleiomorphic rods on micro mean you are dealing with what pathogen? *(popular test item!)*	*H. flu*
What is the most common sequela of meningitis?	**Deafness** (about 10 %)
Which of the typical bacterial meningitides is the mildest?	*Neisseria meningitidis*
When is *Neisseria meningitidis* a highly virulent infection?	**When it is systemic** (bacteremia)
How is H. flu meningitis treated? *(popular test item!)*	**3rd generation cephalosporin** & **Dexamethasone** (give early, before 1st dose of antibiotic if possible)
What is the point of giving dexamethasone with certain forms of meningitis?	It reduces the probability of deafness
If you get a scenario with an H. flu meningitis patient, do household members need any prophylaxis?	**Yes** (Rifampin)

If you need to prophylax a pregnant close contact of a *Neisseria meningitidis* patient, what drug should you use?

Ceftriaxone

If you need to prophylax a non-pregnant adult close contact of a *Neisseria meningitidis* patient, what drug should you use?

Ciprofloxacin
(or rifampin)
(Cipro is a shorter regimen)

The drug of choice for Neisseria meningitis chemoprophylaxis for those <18 years old is _____?

Rifampin

If a patient has a <u>chronic</u> neutrophilic meningitis, what organisms are likely culprits?

(3)

Fungi
Actinomyces
Nocardia

An isolated Bell's palsy, with a chronic meningitis presentation, could be what in a child (or adult)?

Lyme meningitis

What are the most likely causes of aseptic meningitis?

Enterovirus + arboviruses
(enterovirus is most common on the exam)

The medical portion of treating a brain abscess is likely to include what two antibiotics?

Ceftriaxone
       &
Metronidazole (Flagyl®)

What is the most cost-effective way to evaluate a patient for an invasive diarrhea?

Send stool for fecal WBCs

(*popular test item!*)

Thanksgiving, chitlins, and chitterlings, are all associated with what gut infection on the boards?

Yersinia enterocolitica
(pseudoappendicitis presentation)

(*popular test item!*)

When is it not alright to give your patient antimotility drugs for diarrhea?

If you suspect <u>invasive</u> diarrheal illness

Which bacterial causes of diarrhea frequently cause fecal WBCs (invasive disease)?
                    (3)

Shigella
Salmonella
Campylobacter jejuni

Is it alright to treat Salmonella with antibiotics?

Generally, no – greatly increases the chances of becoming a carrier

Which patients are definitely supposed to be treated with antibiotics for Salmonella infection?
                    (3 groups)

The severely immuno-compromised
Children <2 months old
Sickle cell patients

Why is it reasonable to treat certain patient groups for Salmonella diarrhea?

High risk of bacteremia

If a rabbit bite becomes infected, what is the most likely organism?

Pasteurella multocida

(Tularemeia is also theoretically possible, but then there will be a prominent lymph node)

If someone were to get an infection from a pet hamster, what would it be?

(popular test item!)

"Lymphocytic choriomeningitis"

Would that same hamster be a risk to a fetus growing in the same household?

Yes –
The organism is a virus known to cause hydrocephalus, mental retardation, and chorioretinitis with in utero exposure

What is the reservoir for lymphocytic choriomeningitis?

House mice, but it is often transmitted to other wild or domestic rodents

How is lymphocytic choriomeningitis treated?

Supportive care only

(ribavirin may be helpful, but there is no proven treatment)

How is this rodent-related disease transmitted?

Any bodily material from an infected rodent contacting a break in the skin or with inhalation

Name some infections you can catch from your pet ferret? (3)	1. TB 2. Influenza 3. Campylobacter *(Roughly 1 in 5 ferrets have Campylobacter!!!)*

What causes Q fever?

(popular test item!)

Coxiella burnetii

Where is Coxiella burnetii (Q fever) most common in the USA?

(popular test item!)

California

Which animals are the most likely sources for Q fever?

(popular test item!)

Cats

&

Livestock

Biggest concentration of organisms are in the placenta when the animal gives birth

How can you remember the unusual source for some cases of Q fever?

Think of standing in a "queue" to give birth – this reminds you of the placenta

In addition to finding Q fever in placentas, where else do people (especially in vignettes) contract Q fever?

(popular test item!)

Wool & hides –
it survives in tick feces for a year

On micro, a buzzword for Coxiella burnetii is that it is a/an _____ pathogen?

Intracellular

In case you don't remember, due to the astonishingly small number of cases you likely see, what are the symptoms/signs of Q fever?

Mainly flu-like illness
+ diarrhea
+/− pneumonia

When in doubt about the treatment for an unusual disorder on the peds boards, what should your top two choices be?

(Known question of interest)

1. **Tetracycline/doxy-cycline** (≥9 years old)
2. **TMP/SMX**
   (Ciprofloxacin
   in adults)

What is the treatment for Q fever?

Tetracycline

How do you make the diagnosis of Q fever?

Serology

When in doubt, if you are asked how to make a diagnosis on a weird disorder, what should you answer?

Serology

How do you diagnose and treat *Chlamydia psittacci*?

- **Serology**
- **Tetracycline/doxycycline**

A child whose family owns a pet store presents with (mild) tachypnea, cough, & some splenomegaly. You diagnose a pneumonia. Which organism caused it?

(*popular test item!*)

Chlamydia psittaci

(Diagnose by serology, treat with tetracycline or doxycycline)

How exactly do people contract *Chlamydia psittaci*?

Inhaling dried bird excreta

(The birds don't have to be ill appearing)

At a family reunion, most family members come down with a flu-like illness, diarrhea, and some have respiratory symptoms. The family has been eating together, of course, and has also been playing with some kittens that were born during the family gathering. What organism is causing this outbreak?

(*popular test item!*)

Coxiella burnetii
(Q fever)
(the family was exposed to the placenta when the kittens were born)

Why is Augmentin® (Amoxicillin/clavulanate) used for animal bites?

(*popular test item!*)

Because *P. multocida*, the most common pathogen, often has B-lactamase

What dermatologic condition do humans usually acquire from cats?

Ringworm (microsporum canis)

Why would a boards vignette mention that an animal attack (big or small) was "unprovoked?"

(*popular test item!*)

Because they want you to give rabies prophylaxis

Is a vignette that features a cat bite likely to be about rabies, on the boards?	**No –** **Rabies vignettes usually have dog bites, or wild animal contact** (*cats can carry it, though*)
A patient presents with pneumonia and splenomegaly. The vignette mentions birds. What is the organism? (*popular test item!*)	*Chlamydia pstittaci* (Dx: Serology) (Tx: tetracycline/doxy)
If a dog has been fully immunized, then it is immunized against leptospirosis infection. Could a fully immunized dog still give a human leptospirosis?	**Yes –** **Spirochetes can still be excreted in the urine of an immune animal**
How does leptospirosis usually present? (*popular test item!*)	**Jaundice** (no liver necrosis, just dysfunction)
How is leptospirosis diagnosed (let's review)? (*popular test item!*)	**1st week of infection –** **Blood culture** **Later –** **Urine culture** (Tx: PCN or doxy)
Is feline immunodeficiency virus a threat to humans? (*popular test item!*)	**No**
Is feline immunodeficiency virus a threat to severely immunocompromised humans? (*popular test item!*)	**No**
If your cat gets Giardia, are humans in the household at risk to develop it? (*popular test item!*)	**No –** **Not even with immunocompromise** (Imagine a cat with Giardia!)
What is the best way to diagnose a new toxoplasmosis infection?	**IgM**

When during pregnancy is a fetus most likely to become toxoplasmosis infected, if mom catches the infection?

(*popular test item!*)

Mom infected (for the first time) **late in pregnancy**

(the later in pregnancy, the more likely infection is)

Fetal infection with toxoplasmosis is most likely to have *the most severe effects* on the fetus when it happens during what part of gestation?

(*popular test item!*)

Early

Very high eosinophilia and IgG, with a "migratory pneumonia," suggests what possible parasitic infection?

(*popular test item!*)

Visceral larva migrans

(*Toxocara canis* or *cati* worms)

A vignette tells you that a child has a history of <u>pica</u>. The child is now febrile, wheezing, and has developed hepatomegaly. What is the causative organism?

(*popular test item!*)

Visceral larva migrans – Toxocara
(↑eos, ↑IgG, migratory pneumonia)

Other than clinically, how do you make the diagnosis of *Toxocara canis* or cati infection?

ELISA

What is the natural course for toxocara infection?

The worms are in the wrong host, so they die

(spontaneous resolution)

Why would the boards tell you that a child with toxocara has a history of pica?

That's how the child picked up the eggs

Which tapeworm in the really long type?

Pork tapeworm –
4–9 feet!!

Do tapeworms cause problems for humans?

Other than "anal pruritis," not really

How do humans get the short tapeworms? – the kind that infect dogs & cats? From dog/cat fleas

A child from the southern USA is presented on your boards. He has a single coin-shaped or small disc lesion in one of his lungs. What is the lesion, and how should it be treated?

(popular test item!)

- **Dog heartworm (Dirofilaria immitis)**
- **No treatment needed (wrong host)**

Does infection with heartworm produce any symptoms in humans?

(popular test item!)

No –
just the "coin lesion" on CXR, sometimes

How do humans contract heartworm?

(popular test item!)

Mosquito bites

What proportion of people infected with West Nile virus develops *any* clinical symptoms?

(popular test item!)

1 in 5

If a patient develops clinical symptoms of West Nile virus, what are the two possible presentations?

(popular test item!)

1. **Mild flu-like illness** (most patients)
2. **Encephalitis – Hallmark is encephalitis with floppy muscles/low tone**

How do you make the diagnosis of West Nile virus?

Serum IgM

Or

Viral ID from CSF
(RT-PCR test for viral RNA)

An adolescent is presented on your boards. The child is from England, and presents with ataxia and cognitive degeneration. What is the disorder?

(popular test item!)

Mad Cow Disease –
when it affects a person it is called "variant Creutzfeldt-Jakob disease"

What is bovine spongiform encephalopathy?

Mad Cow disease

In addition to ataxia, are other motor changes seen with variant CJD?

(popular test item!)

Yes –

Chorea or myoclonus

What is the characteristic appearance of the brain in new variant CJD?

(popular test item!)

1. **"Florid" plaques** (a lot of plaques)
2. **Spongy changes**

Is the presentation and diagnostic data exactly the same in Creutzfeldt-Jakob and new variant CJD?

No –

The EEG changes are different & presentation tends to be more psychiatric in variant CJD (otherwise they are very much the same)

Have there been cases of variant CJD in the US?

Yes – about 10 –

But all are thought to have caught the disease in England/Great Britain or other areas with bovine spongiform encephalopathy outbreaks

Strep pyogenes belongs to which Strep group?

(popular test item!)

Group A

What is the drug of choice for Strep infection?
(Group A)

(popular test item!)

PCN or Amoxicillin <u>always</u> – there is no resistance

If allergy is an issue, what is an alternative regimen for treating Strep pyogenes?

(popular test item!)

Erythromycin

(or clarithromycin, other macrolides)

If you need to treat a penicillinase resistant organism, what IV "cillin" could you use?

(popular test item!)

Oxacillin/nafcillin

(*Remember, the issue is penicillinase, not methicillin resistance – vanc is <u>not</u> the answer*)

If you are dealing with a β-lactamase resistant organism, what other IV drugs in the PCN family can you still use?

Ampicillin/Sulbactam
Ticarcillin/Clavulanate
Piperacillin/Tazobactam

(*popular test item!*)

What are sulbactam, clavulanate, and tazobactam?

β-lactamase *inhibitors*

(*popular test item!*)

What oral penicillin can be used to fight β-lactamase producing organisms?

Amoxicillin/Clavulanate

(*popular test item!*)

Do all three of the IV PCNs with β-lactamase inhibitors work against pseudomonas?

No –
Ampicillin/Sulbactam does not

(*popular test item!*)

Which oral PCN is effective against pseudomonas?

None!

(*popular test item!*)

What are the main infections that amoxicillin/clavulanate (Augmentin) is good for?
(3)

1. **Bites**
2. **Anaerobes**
3. **Methicillin sensitive Staph aureus & Strep**

(*popular test item!*)

The drug of choice for tularemia is streptomycin, but it is only available in IV form. If your tularemia patient is not sick enough to need IV therapy, what should you use? (Remember, it falls into the weird infections category)

Tetracycline/doxycycline

(*popular test item!*)

What is the treatment for Q fever?

Doxycycline

(*popular test item!*)

What is the treatment for Ehrlichiosis?   Doxycycline

(*popular test item!*)

What is the treatment for Rocky Mountain spotted fever?

(*popular test item!*)

Doxycycline

(chloramphenicol can also be used, if tetracyclines are not available)

Ampicillin is the drug of choice for which two somewhat unusual organisms?

(*popular test item!*)

Listeria

+

Enterococcus (if it is sensitive)

A UTI in a 5-year-old is most likely due to what organism?

(*popular test item!*)

E. coli
(Treat with: TMP/SMX)

If an 18-year-old presents with a UTI, how would you treat him or her?

(*popular test item!*)

TMP/SMX

Or

Ciprofloxacin
(other choices include nitrofurantoin)

If a 1-month-old presents with a UTI, which organisms are you worried about?
(3)

(*popular test item!*)

E. coli
Grp B strep
Listeria

How will you need to treat a 1-month-old with a UTI, initially?

(*popular test item!*)

Ampicillin (for Listeria)

+

Gentamicin or a 3rd-generation cephalosporin

Does ceftriaxone cover pseudomonas?

(*popular test item!*)

No!

A patient is presented who has recently received an antibiotic. History states that the creatinine clearance is impaired. The patient just had a seizure. What are they trying to tell you?

(*popular test item!*)

Reduced creatinine clearance + seizure on antibiotic = <u>imipenem</u>

Which antibiotic should we avoid in the very young due to the (largely theoretical) possibility of biliary sludging? *(popular test item!)*	**Ceftriaxone** (cefotaxime can be substituted)
A child goes swimming in a cow pond and develops amebic meningitis. What is the organism? *(popular test item!)*	**Nigleria**
If you need to treat a *Bordetella pertussis* infection, what is your drug of choice? *(popular test item!)*	**Azithromycin**
What must you always remember about using erythromycin estolate?	**<u>Don't</u> use it in pregnancy**
What is the best & cheapest antibiotic in the aminopenicillin family to treat Enterococcus? *(popular test item!)*	**Ampicillin** (ignore the "amino" part of aminopenicillin)
If Enterococcus creates a bad or severe infection, but it's ampicillin sensitive, what should you do for treatment? *(popular test item!)*	**Treat with ampicillin & gentamicin for synergy**
If Enterococcus is resistant to ampicillin, what should your first antibiotic choice be? *(popular test item!)*	**Vancomycin**
For resistant Enterococcus causing UTI, which medication is often effective?	**Nitrofurantoin!** (avoids using a higher level antibiotic! ☺)
Which infections can still be treated with PCN G or PCN VK? *(popular test item!)*	• **Leptospirosis** • **Meningococcus** (some cases) • **Syphilis** • **Grp A, and often B, Strep infections in the mouth** (developing resistance)

If an IV drug user develops endocarditis, how should you empirically treat it?

(*popular test item!*)

Vancomycin (MRSA)

\+

Gentamicin (synergy + Pseudomonas)

Tobramycin is not really the drug of choice for any infection, except in which category of patients?

(*popular test item!*)

CF patients

(the drug kinetics of tobra in CF patients are very well understood, so it is preferred)

You are worried about possible Pseudomonas infection in a CF patient. You have just started the patient on ceftriaxone for another infection. Will it cover the Pseudomonas?

(*popular test item!*)

No!

A patient on vancomycin develops worsening renal function. Should you consider the vancomycin as a possible cause?

Yes

If your vancomycin patient turns red shortly after you begin infusing vancomycin, what should you conclude?

(*popular test item!*)

It's "red man syndrome" <u>not allergy</u> –

(the whole patient turns red due to histamine dumping by most cells)

Under what conditions will you see "red man syndrome?"

(*popular test item!*)

<u>Rapid</u> infusion of vancomycin

(Slow it down! It's not dangerous, just annoying)

Which ID medications most often cause renal toxicity?

Gentamicin

\+

Amphotericin B

Is it alright to treat a neurotropenic patient with fever with a single drug, if the patient doesn't appear to be particularly ill?

(*popular test item!*)

Yes – <u>if</u>
the drug covers pseudomonas

If a febrile, neutropenic, ill-appearing patient has Gram-negative organisms in the blood, what is the appropriate antibiotic coverage for that patient?

(*popular test item!*)

Two drug therapy –
One to cover pseudomonas and other infections

+

One aminoglycoside for synergy

(**e.g. imipenem + an aminoglycoside, or Timentin® + gentamicin, & sometimes other regimens depending on institution, such a meropenem with fluoroquinolone**)

Which macrolide is associated with transient hearing loss?

(*popular test item!*)

Erythromycin

Which antibiotics target the 50s subunit of bacterial ribosomes?

(*popular test item!*)

Macrolides & oxazolidinones

Lyme disease is usually treated with fairly simple antibiotics such as amoxicillin. If the Lyme disease is very severe, which antibiotic should be used?

(*popular test item!*)

Ceftriaxone

If tobramycin is in the answer choices, you should check the question again, to see whether the patient has what disorder?

(*popular test item!*)

CF

Which oral macrolide has a very long half-life?

Azithromycin

If a patient has both pneumonia and a brain abscess, what is the organism?

(*popular test item!*)

Nocardia
(or occasionally TB)

If a patient has both pneumonia and a brain abscess, what antibiotic will treat the most likely organism?

(*popular test item!*)

TMP/SMX
(Nocardia)

If you are treating a C. diff infection with vancomycin, what <u>must</u> you remember?

(popular test item!)

Vanc will only work if given <u>orally</u>

(Metronidazole works both ways)

Leptospirosis is usually treated with PCN. What other antibiotic is also effective?

Doxycycline/Tetracycline

(of course – it's a "weird infection")

When in doubt, which antibiotic group is most likely to be the cause of ear or kidney damage?

(popular test item!)

Aminoglycosides

What is the "post-antibiotic effect" seen in Gram-negative bacteria?

Gram-negative bacteria die or stop growing even when antibiotic levels drop <u>below</u> the MIC
(Mean Inhibitory Concentration)

Why is the "post-antibiotic effect" important?

Allows once daily dosing of drugs such as aminoglycosides → less renal toxicity

What is a cheap, but good, osteomyelitis treatment? (actually, give the top three!)

1. **Oxacillin**
2. **Cefazolin (Ancef®)**
3. **Clindamycin**

Will ceftriaxone cover Enterococcus?

No
(Ampicillin does)

Can ceftriaxone be used to cover meningococcus?

Yes

Can ceftriaxone cover Listeria?

No –
Ampicillin does!

If Staph aureus is methicillin resistant, will ceftriaxone cover it alright?

No –
Vancomycin does

Is it alright to mix ketoconazole and H2 blockers?

No –
Ketoconazole is only absorbed in an acidic environment

Which medication has coverage very much like an aminoglycoside, plus good Gram-positive coverage, and no renal toxicity?	Aztreonam
Which has better absorption and distribution, PO or IV quinolones?	Equivalent (unless the gut is messed up)
Which special pediatric population with a genetic disorder will need IV quinolones?	CF patients (gut issues)
If a question involves ketoconazole, what is the question likely to be about? *(popular test item!)*	A drug interaction
Is it alright to use ciprofloxacin for a patient already taking theophyllline?	No – the cipro will increase the theophylline level → toxicity
Does cipro provide good coverage for pneumonia?	No – levofloxacin or gatifloxacin do (cipro resistance & Gram-positive coverage is a problem)
You recently started a child on an antibiotic while arranging for a surgeon to evaluate him for appendicitis. The surgeon removed the appendix. Now the boy presents with postsurgical bleeding. What is the problem? *(popular test item!)*	Certain antibiotics impair "recycling" of vitamin K, which can lead to bleeding. (Cefotetan is the most common one)
Antibiotics that impair recycling of vitamin K are most likely to cause bleeding in which patient population?	Those who are already vitamin K deficient
What antibiotic is most likely to cause impaired vitamin K recycling? *(popular test item!)*	Cefotetan

If a patient has a history of a life-threatening anaphylaxis to PCN, is it alright to give a cephalosporin?

(*popular test item!*)

No – the risk is too big if a reaction does occur

What is the probability of a patient reacting to a cephalosporin, if he or she has a PCN allergy?

(*popular test item!*)

2.5 % is the allergy is "confirmed" (1 % if it is a patient reported allergy only)

(This is new data that updates the old wisdom that cross-reactivity is around 10 %)

If a patient has a remote history of an allergic reaction to PCN (such as rash), is it alright to give a cephalosporin on the boards?

(*popular test item!*)

Yes

(*They want you to know both when it is alright, and when you should not take a chance*)

Which cephalosporins have essentially no cross-reactivity with penicillins?

3rd & 4th generation

Which cephalosporins are most likely to cross-react with which penicillins?

Amoxicillin or ampicillin allergy *may* cross-react with:
1st- & 2nd-generation cephalosporins

(has to do with an R-1 side chain the molecules have in common – not with the beta lactam ring)

Can cat scratch disease also be contracted from a cat bite?

Yes (but not as common)

How do humans contract the short (only a few inches) type of tapeworm?

By ingesting infected dog or cat fleas

Dirofilaria, commonly known as heartworm, causes "coin lesions" in human lungs. How is it contracted?

Mosquitoes!

(**same way your dog gets them!**)

What are Osler nodes and what do they indicate?

- **Painful nodules on palms & soles**
- **Subacute bacterial endocarditis**

For visceral larva migrans, when should you consider treatment?

Severe or prolonged symptoms

What <u>is</u> the treatment for visceral larva migrans?	Albendazole
What types of microbes are present in septic abortion?	Polymicrobial – including anaerobes
What significant risks exist for women using the contraceptive sponge? (2)	1. Dislodgement – so it won't work 2. Toxic shock syndrome – if left in place too long
Do spermicides lessen or increase risk of acquiring an STD?	A matter of controversy – it appears that they increase risk of contracting certain disorders and that is the likely boards answer (75 % effective as contraception, when used alone)
Strawberry cervix (little punctuate hemorrhages) and gray-yellow frothy discharge = what diagnosis?	Trichomonas (Treatment: metronidazole or clindamycin)
Slides of your patient's vaginal discharge show something swimming. What is the diagnosis?	Trichomonas
Fishy odor and "clue cells" = what diagnosis?	Gardnerella aka bacterial vaginosis (Treatment: metronidazole or clindamycin)
Do Trichomonas infections require partner treatment to eradicate the infection?	Yes
Is bacterial vaginosis always an STD?	No, but it can be
How do you treat Trichomonas + gardnerella/bacterial vaginosis?	Metronidazole or Clindamycin
Is it okay to use metronidazole in pregnancy?	Not on the boards (ob/gyns sometimes do in early pregnancy though)

Which type of HSV typically affects the genital region?	HSV-2
What are some good techniques for identification of herpes infection? (4)	1. Herpes culture (gold standard) 2. Tzanck test 3. IgG 4. PCR is used with CSF
What is the classic presentation of herpes lesions?	<u>Multiple</u> vesicles (or shallow or crusted erosions), painful and/or itchy
What positive effects will antiviral therapies have on HSV?	1. Shortened episodes 2. Fewer recurrences
For patients with severe or disseminated HSV infection, what should you do?	IV Acyclovir 5–10 mg/kg Q8 hours
Which organism causes syphilis?	Treponema pallidum (a spirochete)
What is the natural course of untreated syphilis?	3 phases: 1 – Single painless skin lesion aka chancre 2 – Rash, especially on palms & soles – darkened macules 3 – Cardiac, ocular, & CNS problems
How is syphilis treated?	PCN
If a pregnant syphilis patient is PCN allergic, what should you use to treat her?	PCN – you will need to desensitize the patient Or Azithromycin (single dose) may be used, but resistance exists, efficacy is lower, & this treatment is not universally accepted (also not by the CDC)
If a syphilis patient does not have any symptoms and the chancre has healed, is s/he likely to be infections?	Yes – at least in the first year after infection

How is the syphilis diagnosis made?	1. RPR or VDRL screening test 2. Confirm with treponemal test
If a patient has been treated for syphilis, will the blood tests for syphilis go back to normal?	Depends – the screening tests usually do, the treponemal tests usually don't
If a nonpregnant patient is PCN allergic, what other med can you use to treat the spirochete?	Doxycycline or Tetracycline (Ceftriaxone is sometimes used, but is less effective & requires 14 days of treatment – not recommended by CDC)
What kind of PCN, specifically, is used to treat syphilis?	Benzathine PCN 2.4 million units IM × 1
If a patient seems to have late-stage or long-term syphilis, what change in the treatment regimen will be needed?	IM PCN every week for 3 weeks
Because some patients fail to respond to PCN treatment of syphilis, what response parameter must be monitored?	Either VDRL or RPR (but you must follow <u>one</u> of them consistently)
What kind of titer response indicates success in treating syphilis?	A 4× drop in VDRL or RPR level
What kind of titer response indicates failure in treating syphilis?	A 4× <u>rise</u> in VDRL or RPR level
Does neurosyphilis only occur with tertiary syphilis?	No – *it can actually occur at any point in the disease*
How is neurosyphilis treated?	IV PCN for 14 days
If a neurosyphilis patient is PCN allergic, what treatment regimen is usually recommended?	Desensitization then PCN (*ceftriaxone is a possible alternative*)
How is neurosyphilis officially diagnosed? (3 components)	CSF VDRL + treponemal tests + clinical signs

What are the clinical signs of neurosyphilis?

(4 groups)

- Meningitis
- Cranial nerve palsies
- Cognitive, motor & sensory deficits
- Eye + ear problems

Syphilis often causes what two ophthalmologic problems?

Iritis and uveitis

A classic boards presentation for neurosyphilis is a young person with _____?

Hearing loss

What unusual reaction sometimes occurs with first-time treatment of syphilis?

Jarisch-Herxheimer (myalgias, fever, chills, back pain)
(especially common in pregnant patients)

A young adult/adolescent presents complaining of eye pain and decreased acuity, bilaterally, with no history of trauma. What diagnosis should you consider?

Uveitis – possibly due to syphilis

Both of the STDs with "granuloma" in the name require 21 days of treatment. What are the two disorders?

- Granuloma inguinale (aka Donovanosis – rare in the US)
- Lymphogranuloma venerum (a special Chlamydia trachomatis infection)

How does Donovanosis (granuloma inguinale) present?

(2 important aspects)

- Painless but *progressive* ulcer
- *No* LAD

How is granuloma inguinale usually treated?

Doxycycline or TMP/SMX for 3 weeks (21 days)

(*longer treatment may be needed if the ulcer or symptoms have not yet resolved – relapses occur up to 18 months after treatment!*)

What is an alternative treatment regimen for granuloma inguinale, in case of allergy or pregnancy?

Macrolides
(erythromycin or azithromycin)

When treating STDs, we often do not do a follow-up culture to prove the cure. Is it necessary to do the follow-up culture if the patient is pregnant?

Yes

Particular types of a common bacterium cause LGV (Lymphogranuloma venerum). What are the types? What is the bacterium?

Serovars (types) L1, L2 and L3 of Chlamydia trachomatis

(*the "L" types cause Lymphogranuloma*)

LGV is uncommon in industrialized nations – why is it important to know about?

(2 reasons)

• It is increasing in industrialized countries
• Failure to treat leads to disfigurement of the genitalia! (& sometimes lymphatic obstruction)
• Failure to treat leads to long term proctocolitis years later!

In which population is LGV especially common?

Men having sex with men

How does LGV present?

A genital ulcer that heals spontaneously and rapidly, then painful unilateral LAD

(The ulcer is often gone before they seek treatment)

How is LGV diagnosed?

Serology

What will get rid of LGV?

21 days of doxycycline or erythromycin

Why is erythromycin <u>estolate</u> contraindicated in pregnancy?

Increased chance of hepatotoxicity

Which STD creates an expanding ulcer that bleeds very easily ("friable surface")?

Donovanosis aka granuloma inguinale

Mnemonic: Use the DIG (Donovanosis Inguinale granuloma) initials to help you remember which one is Donovanosis. DIGgin' a really big ulcer that bleeds

What are the symptoms of urethritis?

Dysuria + urethral discharge

What is the most common cause of "non-gonococcal urethritis?"	Chlamydia
Is it common to have asymptomatic urethritis?	**Yes**
What is the simplest & cheapest way to screen for urethritis?	**Check urine for WBCs – >5/hpf is sensitive and specific for urethritis in males**
What is the usual treatment regimen for urethritis/cervicitis?	Azithromycin 1 g or doxycycline 100 mg BID × 7 days + Ceftriaxone (250 mg once)
Alternative antibiotic regimens, suitable for pregnant (or allergic) patients with STD cervicitis are _____ ? (2)	Erythromycin (500 mg QID × 7 days) Or Amoxicillin (500 mg TID × 7 days) + Ceftriaxone for GC
Otherwise asymptomatic women with cervicitis will sometimes have what symptom after intercourse?	Spotting (of blood)
If a pregnant woman requires treatment for gonorrhea, but she is allergic to cephalo-sporins, how can you treat her?	Azithromycin 2 g in a single dose (*often produces GI distress*)
Is it alright to use quinolones to treat STDs?	No, due to resistance
How is "non-gonococcal urethritis" diagnosed?	If the discharge does not have gram-negative intracellular diplococci, it's called "non-gonococcal"
What recent resistance pattern is developing for *N. gonorrhea*?	Cephalosporin resistance – The recommended dose has been doubled by the CDC! (in 2012 – from 125 to 250 mg IM)
If a patient develops gonorrheal pharyngitis, how would you treat it?	Same as cervicitis

A patient presents with mucopurulent cervicitis and knee pain. She is running a low grade temp. What's the diagnosis?

Gonorrhea (disseminated) with septic arthritis

How is disseminated gonorrheal infection treated?

IV ceftriaxone initially, then PO treatment for at least 1 week (duration depends on problem)

(*other cephalosporin regimens are also approved*)

How does disseminated gonococcus usually present?
(3 options)

1. Skin lesions
2. Right upper quadrant pain (Fitz-Hugh-Curtis Syndrome)
3. Arthritis

Which two vaginal infections raise the pH significantly?
(to >4.5)

Trichomonas

&

Bacterial vaginosis

"Fishy smell" and copious discharge go with which vaginal infection?

Bacterial vaginosis

(sometimes KOH is added to get the fishy odor – usually not necessary)

Sometimes the discharge is not described as "fishy" smelling but rather _____?

"Amine" smelling (bacterial vaginosis)

Recent research shows that treatment of the male partners in cases of bacterial vaginosis is _____?

Not indicated
(*this is a change!*)

If a pregnant woman has bacterial vaginosis, is her pregnancy at risk in any way?

Yes –
Increased risk of preterm labor, PROM, chorioamnionitis

If a pregnant woman develops bacterial vaginosis, how should you treat her?

Clindamycin *PO* –
The cream version actually increases chance of premature birth

(metronidazole is also a possibility but less desirable in pregnancy)

How should you treat pregnant women with Trichomonas infections?

Metronidazole 2 g × one is recommended (even in pregnancy)

(tinidazole is also good for nonpregnant patients)

If you prescribe metronidazole (or other drugs in this class) to an adolescent patient, what do you need to remember to tell the patient?

Drinking alcohol will make them feel very bad!

(Disulfiram-like reaction)

A pregnant patient develops a yeast infection. What is the recommended treatment?

One of the azole creams × 7 days

Frequent candidal vaginitis is a red flag for _____?

HIV infection or diabetes
(*although of course lots of patients with normal immune systems also have this problem*)

What constitutes a treatment failure for outpatient management of PID?

72 hours without clinical improvement

What is the most accepted treatment regimen for Trichomonas?

Metronidazole 500 mg BID × 7 days

(vaginal topical treatment is NOT acceptable due to <50 % cure rate & failure to treat the multiple sites involved!)

If a sexually active woman presents with abdominal pain, but has no abnormal cervical discharge or WBCs on wet prep, what is the likelihood of PID?

Very low

What are two typical regimens for inpatient PID treatment?

Cefoxitin + doxycycline

Or

Clindamycin + gentamicin

(After 24 h of IV therapy with good response, it's okay to change to PO doxy for 14 days)

What is the typical outpatient regimen in pediatrics for PID?	One dose 3rd-generation cephalosporin + Doxycycline × 14 days +/– Metronidazole × 14 days *(metronidazole is for vaginitis, or if there is a recent history of instrumentation)*
How is treatment different if a tuboovarian abscess is also present?	More Gram-negative coverage is needed – Add clindamycin or metronidazole to the regimen
How is the presentation of epididymitis different from that of urethritis?	Epididymitis causes testicular pain/swelling/tenderness
What will <u>symptomatically</u> improve epididymitis?	Pain meds Scrotal elevation/support Bed rest
Epididymitis in an adolescent should be treated how? (<u>different</u> from urethritis)	Ceftriaxone <u>250</u> mg IM + Doxycycline × 10 days
Which types of HPV cause most visible genital warts? (two types)	6 & 11
Which types of HPV are most associated with the later development of cervical cancer and squamous intraepithelial neoplasia (also affecting males)? **(five types)**	**16, 18** **31, 33, and 35**
What are the main treatment modalities for genital warts that can be applied by the patient him or herself? (3)	Podofilox/podophyllin Sinecatechins *(a green tea extract!)* Or Imiquimod
What are the main treatment modalities for genital warts that can only be applied by a medical provider? (3)	• Cryotherapy • Acids (TCA or BCA-types of acetic acid) • Podophyllin resin

Which therapies for genital warts *cannot* be used during pregnancy?
(1 group & 2 specific meds)

- The patient applied types, regardless of who applies them
- Interferon & 5-FU

What complication are infants of women infected with genital wart viruses at risk for?

Laryngeal condyloma
(the virus likes mucosal surfaces, and grows on the larynx, as well)

Is vaginal delivery alright if visible genital warts are present?

Yes –
Unless they directly obstruct delivery

How is genital HPV infection transmitted from mother to infant?

Unknown

Does elective c-section delivery prevent development of laryngeal lesions in the infant?

No

In what percentage of cases of laryngeal papillomatosis due to HPV does the mother have a history of genital HPV?

Just 60 %

Is laryngeal papillomatosis a common problem in at-risk infants?

No –
Only about 2,000 cases per year in the US, despite relatively high HPV infection prevalence

(lesions may develop over first 5 years of child's life)

If you diagnose a subclinical HPV infection, what should you do about it?

Nothing (unless there are squamous intra-epithelial lesons, in which case you follow the usual rules)

If an adolescent is exposed to someone with hepatitis A through sexual contact, what should you do?

Give vaccine or IG
(within *2 weeks* of exposure – long window for efficacy!)

As post-exposure prophylaxis for hepatitis A, which treatment is preferred?

Vaccine, unless –
    Child <1 year old
    Immunocompromise
    Liver compromise
    Or vaccine allergy

If a case of hepatitis A occurs, which *un*immunized persons are considered to be at risk & require prophylaxis?

Household contacts, sexual partners, & illicit drug use partners

Those with "regular" contact, such as babysitters

ALL workers & children at daycare, if children are in diapers

Classroom contacts only if children are not in diapers

If a non-immune patient is exposed to someone with hepatitis B through sexual contact, what should you do?

Give vaccine and IG (different sites, please)

If a patient is exposed to someone with Hepatitis C virus (HCV) through sexual contact, what should you do?

Monitor for seroconversion & hope for the best –
IG doesn't work & there is no vaccine

How should you monitor a patient for development of acute hepatitis C infection?

HCV RNA & liver panel –
The RNA will turn positive significantly earlier than antibody tests!

("*window period*" in which infection is present but antibody is not yet measurable)

If monitoring for hepatitis C indicates that acute infection has begun, what is important to do?

Immediate referral to a specialist for possible early interferon treatment

Scabies is sometimes sexually transmitted. How is it treated?

Permethrin cream (5 %) to whole body from neck down – leave on at least 8 h, then wash off

How does scabies present?

Very itchy patient,
with lines in finger/toe webs & clothing band areas

In order to prevent scabies re-infestation, what additional measures must your patients take?

- Treat other close contacts if they show signs of infection
- Treat bedding/clothing

What organism causes scabies?

Sarcoptes scabiei

Mnemonic:
2nd word sounds like/looks like scabies

Which organism causes pubic lice?   **Pediculosis pubis**

How is pubic lice treated?   Usually lindane or permethrin cream (1 %), just to affected areas

How should you treat a case of pubic lice in a pregnant patient?   Permethrin 1 % cream (NO LINDANE)

Can eyelash lice be treated with permethrin or lindane shampoo/creams?   No – Use topical ophthalmic "occlusive ointments" (in other words, petroleum jelly to suffocate 'em!)

For treatment to be effective, patients with lice will also need to _____?   Decontaminate bedding

Which patients are most likely to develop (infectious) proctitis?   Those who engage in receptive anal intercourse

What are the symptoms of proctitis? (3)   Anorectal pain, discharge, and tenesmus

What are the usual pathogens in sexually acquired infectious proctitis? (4)   *N. gonorrhea* *C. trachomatis* *T. pallidum* HSV

(LGV is also possible)

How is sexually transmitted proctitis treated?   Same as urethritis – Ceftriaxone 250 mg

+

Doxycycline × 7 days (If HSV then acyclovir) (If syphilis then PCN)

How are the symptoms of proctocolitis different from those of proctitis?   The colon is involved, so they have diarrhea and cramps

Are the organisms involved in proctocolitis the same as those involved in proctitis?   No – They are typically invasive diarrheas like Entamoeba or Shigella

Can Giardia be an STD?   Yes, in those who practice oral-anal sex

Which patient group is most often affected in hepatitis E outbreak?   Young males (15–35 years old)

Where are patients most likely to encounter hepatitis E?	In the developing world (also present in the USA, however)
Which patients are at risk for severe hepatitis E infections?	Liver transplant patients & Pregnant women (*20% mortality, worse in 2nd & 3rd trimesters*)
How is hepatitis E mainly spread? (2 ways)	Fecal-oral via water supply & in undercooked pork or deer meat products (*one outbreak reported related to shellfish*)
How serious is hepatitis E infection in children?	Usually mild & self-limited, like hepatitis A
What is the usual course of hepatitis E infection in immunocompetent hosts, in general?	Self-limited
Can hepatitis E infection become chronic?	Yes, in solid organ transplant patients – Otherwise no
Diagnosis of hepatitis E depends on what two tests?	Hep E specific antibodies or HEV RNA
How long after exposure is your patient likely to develop hepatitis E?	40 days! (which means he or she is often back from their trip when they get sick!)
Is there any specific treatment for hepatitis E, or immunization?	No – supportive care only No vaccine in the USA (China has recently made one, but it is not yet approved)
Which hepatitis can *only* infect the liver if the patient is already infected by hepatitis B?	Hepatitis D (the D virus is incomplete – it can't replicate & infant cells without using some of the B virus's machinery)

Is there a vaccine for hepatitis D?

No – but vaccinating against hepatitis B infection will also prevent hepatitis D infection

How serious is hepatitis D infection in an already hep B infected patient?

Serious –
5 % fulminant liver failure

85 % develop chronic hep D infection with increased chance of cirrhosis & hepatocellular carcinoma

What is the best management of hepatitis D, in a patient already infected with hepatitis B?

Monitor for signs of impending liver failure & need for transplant

Interferon treatment for 1 year safe in children, but not very successful in clearing chronic infection

What is the best management of hepatitis D in a patient coinfected with hepatitis B & D at the same time?

Supportive care & monitoring –
Most patients will clear both infections successfully

What is the difficulty with a positive serological test for Lyme disease?

It tells you whether the patient was exposed, but not whether she or he is currently infected (antibodies are present for a long time)

&

Antibody tests are often negative in early acute infection!

Which sign of Lyme disease means you should treat empirically, without further laboratory confirmation?

Erythema migrans
(with reasonable risk of exposure to ticks)

If your patient does *not* have an erythema migrans rash, but you still suspect Lyme disease, what should you do to confirm it?

2-step process:
ELISA or IFA, if positive

Do Western blot

Treat only if both are positive!

(IFA = immunofluorescence assay)

Does small pox occur naturally?

No – it is completely eradicated. If you see it, it is bioterror
(or a similar appearing related disorder)

How is small pox treated?

Supportive care only + quarantine to prevent spread

What limits immunization of the population against small pox? (we did it before . . .)

Significant cardiotoxicity occasionally occurs

&

Disseminated disease is more likely now due to prevalence of immunocompromise & certain skin disorders

How do small pox patients present?

Ill appearing (severe flu-like illness), with diffuse blistering on mucous membranes & external skin
Lesions are *all in the same stage* & diffusely present on the body

Is small pox uniformly fatal?

No –
Around 40 % overall

(30 % for the most common type, 95 % for the two worst types but these develop in only about 5 % of the patients)

How easily does small pox spread? Will everyone in a crowd get it, if an infected person walks through?

Fairly easily, but it usually requires close face-to-face or bodily fluid contact

Contact with contaminated items like bedding can spread the disease

Only *rarely spread* via air in *enclosed* spaces

Contagious small pox patients are also usually quite ill & not likely to be walking far!

What relatively common infectious diseases sometimes cause AV block?
(2)

Viral myocarditis

&

Lyme disease

(some zebras, too, such as Chagas disease)

Does JIA (juvenile idiopathic arthritis) cause valvular heart disease?

No – it can cause myocarditis/ pericarditis

What are the most common & well-known infectious causes of myocarditis?

Coxsackie A & B viruses (especially Coxsackie B)

(Coxsackie viruses are enteroviruses)

Recent PCR-based studies have showns that which two other viruses are currently very common causes of myocarditis?

HHV 6 (virus associated with roseola infantum)

&

Parvovirus B19

Historically, which two viruses were thought to cause most myocarditis (& still do cause it regularly)?

Adenoviruses

&

EBV

Is viral myocarditis, the most common type of myocarditis in children, a common problem?

No –
For example, only about 2 % of patients with
enteroviral infection develop myocarditis

What physical findings are noted in myocarditis?

CHF findings, and *no murmur*

If a myocarditis patient has pulsus paradoxus, what would that make you think?

Possible pericardial effusion (causing tamponade)

How do you document a diagnosis of viral myocarditis?

Viral serology & cultures

What is the main goal of myocarditis treatment, in terms of cardiac tissue?

Minimize hemodynamic demands to minimize cardiac tissue damage

Which myocarditis patients require inpatient treatment?

Any with symptoms –
Decompensation can occur rapidly!

Are blood-borne parasites known to cause myocarditis?

Yes –
Lyme, Babesiosis, &
Ehrlichiosis all can
(not often, though)

Which two bacteria are most often involved in the uncommon *bacterial* myocarditis?

Corynebacterium diphtheriae (diphtheria)

&

Staph aureus

Are myocarditis cases always due to infectious causes?

No –
Drugs, toxins, hypersensitivity and other reactions can cause it

How bleak is the prognosis in pediatric myocarditis?

It depends on the cause, but complete recovery may occur in up to 50 % of cases

Index

Printed by Printforce, the Netherlands